ENDOMETRIOSIS

"The doctor shoved a book in my face and went off to talk on the phone. I thought I had some kind of cancer! Later, I looked up endometriosis in a medical dictionary and found out that it was a condition in which the tissue of the uterus attaches to other organs."

"I didn't realize the seriousness of the problem, especially regarding difficulty in pregnancy and later need for hysterectomy. For all I knew, it could have been a name for bad breath or fallen arches, because he [the doctor] made it seem so minor."

"Each month the pain came earlier and earlier until I hurt ten days before my period started. My doctor said it was my imagination."

"My family and boyfriend are all supportive of me, but I don't think they'll ever understand how this condition can severely limit my schedule."

"I have suffered from this disease for approximately two-and-a-half years, but I'm sure it went undetected for many years before this."

"If I had decided to get pregnant, would my unborn child be affected by the disease? I feel so ignorant on the subject."

"If I had anything to tell other women, it would be that they should observe everything about endometriosis, look at all the alternatives."

"My doctor told me to get pregnant and I don't even have a boyfriend!"

"It's as though you selfishly brought endometriosis on yourself because you delayed having children."

"My husband and I could have flown to Maui and back many times on what I spent on doctors' bills, tests, and pills as costly as rubies."

"All our years of searching, all the frustrations of misdiagnosis, all the pain of surgery ended in success. Today, we have a child."

"They finally did a laparoscopy and discovered I had endometriosis. I was put on birth control pills. [Now] I have two beautiful children. For those eight years I considered myself cured. Wrong. I am again going through the pain and misery."

"I hated the danazol, and the emotional swings were murder—and I hated my body after putting on thirty pounds. The danazol was effective, however."

"I had a severe case of endometriosis. My doctor-surgeon was able to burn or scrape some adhesions and following surgery she began comprehensive treatment with Danocrine. On my most recent visit . . . she could find no traces remaining."

"It involves your feelings about being a woman, about sexuality and infertility. There is a lot of real, deep pain around infertility."

"You lose your sense of who you are. You lose sight of your dreams—you can't plan things anymore."

Also by Julia Older

ENDOMETRIOSIS

Julia Older

Foreword by Anne B. Ward, M.D.

MACMILLAN • USA

For my mother, Louise Dalrymple Older, and my sisters, Debbie Hall and Priscilla Older.

Copyright © 1984 Julia Older

Material from *Patient Care* magazine copyright © 1978, Patient Care Communications, Inc., Darien, Conn. All rights reserved. Reprinted by permission of the publisher.
Figure 1 on p. 4 is used with the permission of the Syntex Corporation, Palo Alto, Calif.
Figures for classification of endometriosis from R. W. Kistner, "Endometriosis" in *Gynecology and Obstetrics*, ed. John Sciarra (Hagerstown, Md.: Harper & Row, 1980), Chap. 38. Reprinted by permission of the publisher.

Macmillan General Reference
A Simon & Schuster Macmillan Company
1633 Broadway
New York, NY 10019-6785

Library of Congress Cataloging-in-Publication Data

Older, Julia, 1941–
  Endometriosis.

  Includes bibliographical references and index.
  1. Endometriosis.   I. Title.   [DNLM: 1. Endometriosis—
Popular works.   WP 903 044e]
RG483.E53043   1984   618.1'42   83-20824
  ISBN 0-684-18505-9

10

Printed in the United States of America

ACKNOWLEDGMENTS

MANY PEOPLE HAVE contributed their time, knowledge, and skills toward the publication of this book. Not least among them have been the women who participated in interviews, often sharing painful and disheartening problems. Their participation has not only encouraged the author, but will be invaluable to others.

My appreciation goes to Drs. George T. Schneider, Malcolm Potts, Robert W. Kistner, Paul D. Manganiello, Anne B. Ward, John A. Rock, John C. Weed, John Herbert Niles, Michael Osterholm, and the many other physicians and researchers who have generously shared their views on endometriosis.

I would especially like to thank my editor, Susanne Kirk, and my agent, Martha Millard, for their enthusiastic support in all aspects of this project.

Special thanks are extended to Mary Lou Ballweg of the Endometriosis Association for her assistance and involvement in the compilation of material, and to Dr. Anne Ward for reviewing the manuscript.

The cooperation of personnel at the Francis A. Countway Library of Medicine of Harvard, and especially the staff of the rare book room, is most gratefully acknowledged. In addition, I want to thank John Bundy at the Dana Biomedical Library of Dartmouth, and the always helpful librarians of the Peterborough Town Library, Peterborough, New Hampshire. I am also indebted to Eve Nichols for her information search at Tufts University, and to Phyllis T. Piotrow, director of the Johns Hopkins Population Information Program, for her POPLINE search.

Several private and government institutions have contributed information to this book. Among them are: International Fertility Research Program, Winthrop Laboratories, The American Fertility Society, Syntex Laboratories, U.S. Food and Drug Administration, International Planned Parenthood Federation, Public Health Service (HEW), and many others. It is difficult to thank all the contributors, but I would like to emphasize their input.

I offer special thanks to all my friends for their suggestions, clippings, contacts, and continued interest.

Above all, I wish to express my appreciation (and sympathy) to Steve Sherman, who patiently lived through ENDOMETRIOSIS, listened, proofread, and often placed this book before his own work. His inspiration was mine.

Contents

Foreword   xiii

Preface   xv

PART ONE
THE CONDITION

1. *Endometriosis: Women and Life Decisions*   3
    Were You Meant to Have 425 Periods—or 50?   5
    Insulting the Peritoneum   8

2. *The Endometrium and Endometriosis*   10
    Menstrual Backup (The Retrograde
      Menstruation Theory)   10
    Blood and Lymph Glands (Transplantation
      Theory)   12
    Nosocomial Infection (Accidental Implantation)   13
    Invasion of the Uterus (Adenomyosis)   15

3. *More a Condition Than a Disease*   18
    Antibodies (The Immunologic Theory)   19
    Hormone Levels (Hormonal Imbalance)   21
    The Benign Cancer (Transformation)   22
    Family Connections (Genetic Predisposition)   24

4. *Symptoms*   26
Common Complaints   27
A Symptom Sampler   31
Choosing a Doctor   36
Disease with Similar Symptoms   38

5. *Infertility: A Major Symptom*   44
The Infertility Workup   44
Being Classified   49
Chances of Fertility   50
The Therapeutic Baby   56

PART TWO

TREATMENTS

6. *Laparoscopy and Other Methods for Diagnosis*   61
"Let's Wait and See"   62
Laparoscopy and Biopsy   66
Chocolate Cysts and Powder Burns   72
Ultrasound   74

7. *Medical Treatment: Hormones*   77
Pseudopregnancy (Combination Hormones)   78
Pseudomenopause (Danazol)   85

8. *Surgery: Conservative or Radical?*   92
Evaluating Priorities   92
A Second and Third Opinion   93
How Conservative?   96
What to Expect   96
Nothing Is Routine   99
Microsurgery   102
How Radical?   104

9. *Radiation Therapy*   108

10. *Rare Complications*   112
Ovarian Endometriosis and Ovarian Cancer   112
Endometriosis of the Bowel   113
Endometriosis of the Lung   114

Endometriosis of the Navel and Other Strange
    Sites   114

PART THREE
THE FUTURE

11. *Endometriosis in Teenagers*   119
    The Cause   120
    Early Diagnosis and Treatment   121

12. *Menopause: Home Free?*   126
    Hormones and Menopause   127
    Coping with Premature Menopause   129
    Adenomyosis   130

13. *The Career Woman's Disease: Fact or Fantasy?*   133
    Somatotype   134
    Personality   136
    Socioeconomic Status   138
    A Need for Statistics   140
    The Making of a Myth   144

14. *Race: Turning the Tables*   146
    Black Women   147
    Jewish Women   150
    Oriental Women   152

15. *Prevention*   155
    Early Detection   156
    Correction of Genital Abnormalities   157
    Tampons Versus Sanitary Pads   159
    Sexual Intercourse During Menstruation   160
    IUD and Cervical Cap Wearers   162
    Pelvic Studies and Surgical Procedures
        Performed During Menstruation   163
    Beneficial Aspects of the Pill   164
    An Ounce of Prevention Is Worth a
        Seven-Pound Baby   166
    Menstrual Extraction   167
    Nutrition   168
    Addendum   170

16. Leeches and Laudanum: Grandmother and You   171
    Historical Highlights   171
    Great-Great Grandmother   173
    Great-Grandmother   177
    Grandmother and Mother   180
    You   180

Appendix A   182

Appendix B   184

Glossary   188

Bibliographical Notes   196

Index   215

Foreword

I FIRST BECAME interested in endometriosis as an obstetrics-gynecology (ob-gyn) resident in training. One of my mentors, with whom I was later associated in private practice for several years, became almost obsessed with proving that black as well as white women suffered from this disease, although all the gynecological textbooks claimed the contrary. He subsequently published an article in one of the ob-gyn journals about his findings. Because of his virtual crusade at our hospital, I and several others began to look for the disease in women who complained of chronic pain. *And we found it!*

We now know that endometriosis spares no race or nationality, that women who have careers as homemakers are just as prone to this problem as are women executives who have postponed childbearing. In my own private practice I have identified endometriosis in women of various racial and ethnic backgrounds—black, Polish, Jewish, Puerto Rican, Mexican, Italian, and a Fiji Islander, to list a few. As laparoscopy becomes a more common procedure in developing countries, more endometriosis is being found.

Endometriosis is also not just a disease of women in their thirties. Dr. Donald L. Chatman and I have reported our findings in adolescents complaining of pelvic pain. The youngest patient reported in the literature that I am aware of was nine years old. I have seen one thirteen-year-old girl, and several between ages thirteen and nineteen, with documented endometriosis.

Another very interesting aspect of this disease is that there may be an entity we (Dr. Chatman and I) call "emerging endometriosis." We applied this term to cases in which all the symptoms and physical findings strongly suggested endometriosis, but, when the patient underwent laparoscopy, no obvious endometrial lesions could be visualized. I know of at least three patients who qualify for this diagnosis, having undergone two or even three laparoscopic procedures by the same physician, where initial assessment of the pelvic organs was negative, and the second or third assessment showed obvious evidence of disease. I would strongly recommend to women who suffer from chronic pelvic pain and who have been told that laparoscopic findings were negative: if the pain continues or worsens despite various treatments, a second laparoscopy may be strongly indicated.

When I was asked to review the manuscript for this book, I did so with enthusiasm. Not much has been written for the lay person about endometriosis; there are really no comprehensive sources of information about this disease available. The book is filled with information, and actually goes far beyond the scope of endometriosis alone; the basis of much of the female endocrinological apparatus is explained fully and simply. This book will have many applications, not only for women trying to cope with the problems and consequences of endometriosis, but for all women who would like to understand their reproductive functions.

Anne B. Ward, M.D., F.A.C.O.G.

Preface

WHEN MY GYNECOLOGIST told me that he would like to perform a laparoscopy to rule out possible problems including endometriosis, I agreed. I knew about endometriosis (en-dō-mēt-ri-ōs'-əs) because my mother had suffered from it. As it turns out, I did not have endometriosis, but by then my curiosity was aroused.

Whenever I explained to friends why I was going into the hospital, they would grow animated and say, "Oh, I have a friend who nearly died from it," or "I had it, you know. I finally had to have a hysterectomy." Their reactions were unusually strong.

So I decided to do some basic reading about the condition. One of the first articles I read was a personal account in a popular magazine. The author said that she could not find one book on endometriosis. She added, "This made me believe that doctors really don't know much about endometriosis; someone would have written a book about it."

Surely she must be wrong, I thought. In my own small circle of friends, at least one out of four knew about the condition, or had it themselves. I checked *Books in Print*, but did not find one entry for endometriosis. The author had been correct. Next, I checked health encyclopedias and women's health guides. Many of them allotted endometriosis one short paragraph, if that. A few of the more recent gynecologic guides for women expanded the information to a short chapter at most.

In a more thorough investigation at Harvard's Francis A. Countway Library of Medicine, one of the largest in the country, my initial search yielded only one medical text devoted to endometriosis, and that was written in Spanish!

Thus, my journey began. I started to unravel the popular myths and wind through the labyrinth of contradictory information amassed by doctors over the last decades. I discovered that whereas popular articles on endometriosis numbered a handful, the *Index Medicus* listed hundreds of articles, especially in the last few years.

But how many women would have access to a medical library to learn about their particular case of endometriosis? Once again, I realized how true the maxim is that knowledge is power. Women learn from most popular magazine and newspaper articles that endometriosis is a mysterious condition that usually affects white, egocentric, career-oriented, childless women in their late twenties. Doctors investigating the numerous articles listed in the *Index Medicus* learn much more. They evaluate data on endometriosis that explore every single detail of the condition from the accidental implantation of endometriosis in surgical scars to the incidence found in teenagers.

The reaction of women who discovered I was writing this book took on even greater force. At casual gatherings, when asked the usual "What are you working on?" I learned to reply evasively, "A women's health book." This response was for self-protection after being approached many times by women who had endometriosis or thought they had it. In a rush, they would be upon me asking if this were true or if I could explain that. While other guests talked about the state of the economy and foreign policy, we talked of retroverted uteri and menstrual cramps.

It is for those women that this book has been written, for all those women who have wanted to ask questions for so long. Even if the answers are not always clear, I believe that just being informed enough to ask the right questions will serve a purpose. No doubt, some women might disagree with the conclusions of certain studies. Possibly, doctors will disagree with what other doctors have written or said. What matters, however, is to present the many viewpoints, the controversial theories and contradictory data, so that women everywhere may at least have access to it.

Although I escaped endometriosis, my mother was less fortunate. Her youth was plagued by monthly pain, and the difficulties of her early married life were exacerbated by the pressure to have her family as quickly as possible. She "lost" years of her life incapacitated by the disease.

While writing the section on family connections (see pp. 24–25), it suddenly dawned on me that I should find out whether either of my sisters showed my mother's susceptibility. Sure enough, one sister (with two children) confided that a few endometriosis implants had been accidentally discovered and removed during surgery for another condition. My younger sister suffered from infertility problems before having her two children. Infertility is a known symptom of endometriosis. It is ironic that I escaped endometriosis; supposedly, I was the intentionally childless, egocentric, career-minded member of the family.

I have attempted to set down information without bias. Sometimes that has been difficult, because women and their doctors often do not see eye to eye. Nonetheless, it is my fervent hope that this book will spark a long-needed dialogue —not a monologue or a diatribe, but an honest interchange of views—through which the doctor and patient may arrive at the best possible solutions.

J. O.

PART ONE

THE CONDITION

1

Endometriosis: Women and Life Decisions*

To UNDERSTAND HOW endometriosis works, it is first necessary to review the familiar cyclical process that takes place in a woman's body from puberty to menopause.

During menstruation, the lining of the uterus (endometrium) becomes engorged (swollen) with blood to prepare for possible conception. This activation of the blood vessels and glands is set off by the secretion of the female sex hormones estrogen and progesterone from the ovaries. The lining of the uterus must be prepared for the fertilized egg. In fact, whether or not the egg is fertilized, the lining becomes soft and thick with tissue and may thicken ten times by mid-cycle. On approximately the fourteenth day, counting from day one of the last menstrual period, the egg is released from the ovary. If it is not fertilized by sperm and the woman is not pregnant, the female sex hormone levels decline. Then the endometrial tissue of the uterus breaks down and menstruation occurs, flushing blood and tissue out the vagina. A new cycle starts. If conception does occur, the fertilized egg

---

*For full information on sources referred to throughout this book, see the bibliography on page 196. Terms not defined in the text may be found in the Glossary on page 188.

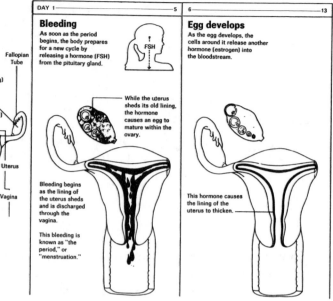

Pituitary Gland

Fallopian Tube

Ovum (mature egg)

Ovary

Ovary (inside)

Uterus

Vagina

Cervix

DAY 1 — 5

Bleeding

As soon as the period begins, the body prepares for a new cycle by releasing a hormone (FSH) from the pituitary gland.

FSH

While the uterus sheds its old lining, the hormone causes an egg to mature within the ovary.

Bleeding begins as the lining of the uterus sheds and is discharged through the vagina.

This bleeding is known as "the period," or "menstruation."

6 — 13

Egg develops

As the egg develops, the cells around it release another hormone (estrogen) into the bloodstream.

This hormone causes the lining of the uterus to thicken.

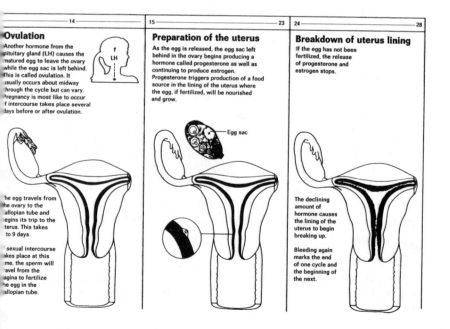

14 —

Ovulation

Another hormone from the pituitary gland (LH) causes the matured egg to leave the ovary while the egg sac is left behind. This is called ovulation. It usually occurs about midway through the cycle but can vary. Pregnancy is most like to occur if intercourse takes place several days before or after ovulation.

LH

The egg travels from the ovary to the fallopian tube and begins its trip to the uterus. This takes to 9 days.

sexual intercourse akes place at this me, the sperm will avel from the agina to fertilize he egg in the allopian tube.

15 — 23

Preparation of the uterus

As the egg is released, the egg sac left behind in the ovary begins producing a hormone called progesterone as well as continuing to produce estrogen. Progesterone triggers production of a food source in the lining of the uterus where the egg, if fertilized, will be nourished and grow.

Egg sac

24 — 28

Breakdown of uterus lining

If the egg has not been fertilized, the release of progesterone and estrogen stops.

The declining amount of hormone causes the lining of the uterus to begin breaking up.

Bleeding again marks the end of one cycle and the beginning of the next.

attaches to the protective fleshy wall of the uterus, eventually forming the placenta that sustains the fetus.

In many women of reproductive age, however, some of the endometrial tissue ordinarily expelled from the body through menstruation travels outside the uterus and sticks there. In susceptible women, this tissue implants itself on the ovaries, the Fallopian tubes, the outer wall of the uterus, the pelvic lining, the cervix, or the vagina. This condition is known as endometriosis.

Endo is a Greek word meaning within, and *metri* refers to the Greek *metra*, or uterus. *Osis* is a suffix that means an abnormal or diseased condition. Put them all together and you have "an abnormal condition within the uterus."

In fact, the problem lies outside the uterus. Emigrating endometrial tissue implants itself on other organs. The grafted patches of endometrial tissue, although most commonly localized in or near the reproductive system, have been found in the rectum, on the intestine, on the appendix, and as far away as the elbow.

Acting as though they were still in the uterus, these refugee endometrial cells respond every month to the same hormones produced during the menstrual cycle. So although they are exiled from their uterine home, they thicken, enlarge, and bleed as if they were still inside the uterus. If the woman is lucky, these misplaced endometrial enclaves are not situated near nerve endings, and may not cause any pain at all. Otherwise, they can, and often do, make her life miserable.

WERE YOU MEANT TO HAVE 425 PERIODS—OR 50?

If a woman with endometriosis stops menstruating, the endometrial tissue that forms cysts and implants does not engorge, does not cause subsequent lesions, and in fact remains inactive. Growing evidence shows that endometriosis is much less common in countries where women menstruate fewer times. In these countries, the onset of menstruation occurs later, childbearing begins earlier, breast-feeding is prolonged, and menopause starts prematurely by our standards.

Dr. Malcolm Potts, Executive Director of the International Fertility Research Program, thinks that endometriosis begins with the whole phenomenon of menstruation. "I think that women probably have menstrual periods because in biological terms human beings are rather inefficient," he observes. "If a woman does not get pregnant, the uterus goes back to a state where she can ovulate again. Menstruation speeds up that process by allowing the tissue to shed and grow again, rather than reorganizing it. Certainly, it doubles the blood requirements and is a very curious process. There are only a few species of animals that menstruate, and they're all relatively slow breeders."

Dr. Potts refers to the Kung bush women of the Kalahari Desert in Botswana, South Africa. Many sociological studies have centered on these people. In primitive tribes, the women menstruate fairly late compared to our average twelve-and-a-half years. (Our grandmothers' average menarche, or first menstrual period, appeared at fourteen years of age.) Many tribal women become pregnant in their teens and breast-feed their children from two to four years before weaning. This could add up to nearly five years without the interruption of a menstrual period. This pattern continues until early menopause. Menstruation can become very rare—at most fifty periods.

In developed countries, on the average, women have their first children in their twenties. By the age of twenty-one, a woman can already have experienced about ninety menstrual periods. If she has two children, does not breast-feed, and reaches menopause at fifty years of age, she may have had a total of 425 menstrual periods! Dr. Potts concludes, "The whole pattern of menstruation has been altered by civilized living."

Today, women might well argue that breast-feeding an infant for several years just to avoid menstruation would be unnatural. Most researchers in fertility and reproduction tend to agree. They do point out, however, that the woman's reproductive system did evolve around lactation and breast-feeding as a means for a natural, built-in contraceptive.

Dr. Roger Short, currently Professor of Reproductive Biology at Monash University, Australia, addresses the long-term problem confronting societies. He believes that we have tackled the dilemma of birth control illogically and irrationally. "We must ask ourselves some critical questions," Dr. Short writes. "What is the optimal state of repose for a uterus that we no longer need to produce babies, an ovary that is no longer required to ovulate, and breasts that we do not want to produce milk? Only when we have answered these questions will we be in a position to offer women what they deserve, namely, healthy fertility."

What has all this to do with endometriosis? The answer lies in Dr. Short's reference to healthy fertility. Except for fibroid tumors, endometriosis has been reported as the most common cause for infertility in the United States, and in most other developed countries as well.

A serious problem exists to be resolved. The first step rests with women and a confident new approach to the dissemination of literature about their own bodies. The second step is for all of us to realize that we live in a world that makes great demands on the human body. Whether or not women agree with the doctors and researchers, they must confront the increasing problems associated with modern living. As one Boston woman interviewed put it, "Endometriosis is bound up with social and emotional unrest. It's all bound up with the 'life decisions' such as pregnancy and marriage."

Until now, many solutions have proven less than satisfactory. Some women's breasts become tender when they are on high-estrogen pills because the Pill simulates pregnancy without resultant suckling. The intrauterine device (IUD) often does not keep the uterus in a healthy state. As Dr. Potts commented in an interview for this book, "The whole pattern of repeated menstruation is not what Charles Darwin intended. I think it's reasonable to speculate that eventually we would develop a hormone medication that would put the body into a state resembling pregnancy and lactation without the baby and the milk. I think it would cut down on breast cancer, endometriosis, and fibroids. It would act as an artificial means to put a woman back into a natural situation."

INSULTING THE PERITONEUM

One of the leading doctors in the treatment of endometriosis in infertile women is Dr. Robert W. Kistner of the Harvard Medical School and Brigham and Women's Hospital in Boston, Massachusetts. He looks at the problem from a closer perspective, usually through the lens of a diagnostic tool called the laparoscope. As a specialist, he often sees up to thirty women in his office in one day. They come to him from around the world, and most of them suffer from infertility because of endometriosis.

Dr. Kistner remembers one woman who came to him several years ago. She was forty-two years old and had endometriosis, but had recently decided that she wanted to get pregnant. "The chances of her getting pregnant with extensive endometriosis at forty-two years of age were zero," he said. "You see, for thirty years she'd been insulting her peritoneum."

The peritoneum is a delicate membrane that lines the abdominal and pelvic cavities and covers the organs that lie within them. As we have noted, endometrial tissue becomes implanted on this lining, causing cysts and subsequent scarring, which are irritated by monthly menstruation. A thirty-year period of uninterrupted activity of this nature not only interferes with normal childbearing, but can interfere with the body processes as a whole.

A book on endometriosis should not try to convince women that a family might be cheaper (and healthier) by the dozen. Nor should it attempt to persuade her to take artificial sex hormones or to have her uterus and ovaries removed. Insulting the peritoneum is not life-threatening in medical terms. One rarely dies from endometriosis.

We cannot escape the twentieth century. But we can consider our own priorities in respect to the outside world and in relation to the intimate and innate system of our bodies. Let us hope that women will take the initiative. Even if it is too late for our generation, at least we may begin to explain to our daughters the physiological consequences that sometimes accompany certain life decisions.

These are facts that girls should be told, not just at puberty (and many are socially and psychologically prime before their time) but before, when questions arise about menstruation. Item: By the age of thirty-five to thirty-nine years, their chances for pregnancy will have decreased by 20 percent. Item: Endometriosis is the leading cause of infertility in women in their twenties. In approximately 40 to 50 percent of these cases, the infertility will be permanent. Item: Long periods of ovulation without interruption (for whatever reason) can predispose women to endometriosis.

If these important considerations are explained to twelve- and thirteen-year-olds in tandem with the facts of life, fewer women tomorrow will suffer from pain, the adverse side effects of medical and surgical treatment, and the sometimes irreversible damage to their reproductive systems.

Early information and knowledge will help women to recognize endometriosis and will assist them in choosing the direction of their lives without fear. For the first time in 150 years, the facts about endometriosis have become available. Facts concerning endometriosis are open for discussion, questioning, and exploration, not only by the medical profession, but by us—our daughters, our sisters.

2

The Endometrium and Endometriosis

IN THE 1920S, researcher John Sampson coined the word *endometriosis*. Sampson described several theories about processes that might lead to endometriosis, but he supported the reflux or retrograde menstruation theory as the most probable cause. Since then, more than a dozen other suppositions have waxed and waned, with most research substantiating and adding to the validity of Sampson's initial proposal.

Unfortunately, although the "how" of endometriosis has been narrowed down to three or four likely explanations, the "why" lags far behind.

MENSTRUAL BACKUP
(The Retrograde Menstruation Theory)

Simply stated, this theory proposes that endometrial tissue from the uterus backs up and out the Fallopian tubes and into a woman's abdominal cavity. Dr. Robert Kistner, the Harvard Medical School specialist, emphasizes, however, that "every woman pushes blood out through her [Fallopian] tubes every month." Through laparoscopy performed during a woman's menstrual cycle, Dr. Kistner and others have observed menstrual blood in the tubes of scores of women. Sampson's retrograde menstruation theory may still be correct, but in 1922 the fact that *every* woman loses some menstrual blood through her Fallopian tubes had not yet been proven, and today seeing is believing.

Many health writers seem unaware of this recent discovery and make statements such as the following from an article on endometriosis syndicated in the *Los Angeles Times:* "It is theorized that during menstruation, fragments of endometrial tissue may back out through the Fallopian tubes and collect on pelvic organs." This statement is misleading because it intimates that only in a few women do these endometrial fragments back out through the tubes. Evidence substantiates the fact that *all* women show some retrograde bleeding. What is perplexing is that in some women the tissue tends to "collect on pelvic organs."

In effect, researchers have begun to conclude that finding endometrial fragments outside the uterus is actually quite common. The fact that in some women it "sticks" is not.

Experiments have been conducted on female monkeys in which the uterus was turned upside down so that the cervix, or mouth of the uterus, projected inside the abdominal cavity. Blood from the menses would spill into the cavity instead of out the vagina. Six out of ten monkeys developed endometriosis.

Some doctors believe that endometriosis is linked to the *amount* of menstrual blood pushed through the tubes. The monkey experiments show that if all the menstrual blood is dumped into the peritoneal cavity, endometriosis develops in about 60 percent of the cases. Still, the question arises: Why do 40 percent remain untouched by the condition?

In one of the few medical textbooks devoted completely to endometriosis, author J. A. Chalmers, M.D., asserts that many doctors agree that the obstruction—for whatever reason—of menstrual flow also plays a part in the causes of the condition.

Opinions differ from doctor to doctor, however, and much of the research material confuses the issue. Some doctors are convinced that a retroverted or tipped uterus exacerbates endometriosis by causing more backup, and others emphatically deny that the position of the uterus has anything to do with the menstrual flow, unless the uterus is in a permanently frozen position. (The uterus can be plastered by endometrial implants into a fixed position.) In opposition, some researchers working with teenage women have found that very few of the cases show genital abnormalities causing blockage.

Another theory advanced by a few practitioners asserts that retrograde menstruation is actually caused by primary spasmodic dysmenorrhea (menstrual cramps occurring the first day of the period). They suggest that these muscular spasms of the uterus force the menstrual blood to gush up through the Fallopian tubes.

Pretend we are researchers tracking down the culprit of endometriosis. Our sleuthing thus far has led us to surmise that endometriosis is caused by an abundant menstrual backup from the Fallopian tubes into the peritoneal cavity.

Yet cases have been found in the armpits, the lungs, and the groin as well. Even if these cases prove the exception, how did the endometriosis get to these sites? The retrograde menstruation theory takes the tissue as far as the peritoneal cavity and no farther. Perhaps to discover how the ectopic (misplaced) tissue travels to distant sites, we must follow another trail.

BLOOD AND LYMPH GLANDS
(Transplantation Theory)

Sampson was able to recognize endometrial tissue in the blood and lymph glands. The process of transference from one place to another via these channels is referred to as metastasis. He concluded that his discovery did not necessarily invalidate the retrograde menstruation theory.

Consider a dandelion gone to seed. The seed may be borne by the wind and transported to a neighboring yard. Or perhaps it sticks to the fur of a dog who trots to a neighboring yard and rolls in the grass; the dog transplants the seed. Or the seed could blow onto a passing windshield and be carried across three states. The analogy should be clear. There is more than one way to disseminate a dandelion seed. The same might be true of endometriosis.

Endometrial lesions have been found in regional lymph nodes. Lymph nodes act as a filter to eliminate unwanted cells from the lymph fluid, providing a sort of runoff for the uterus and other pelvic structures to drain into. Lymph nodes are strategically placed in the lymph gland system. Some are located in the armpit. Although rare, endometriosis has been found in the armpit. It has also been discovered in lymph nodes and the inguinal canal of the groin.

Researchers have recognized that the lymph theory tends to answer certain questions—for example, how endometrial tissue gets into the pleura (lining) of the lungs. A few unfortunate women with endometriosis cough up blood during their menstrual cycles.

Blood and lymph circulate throughout the body and may prove to be carriers of endometrial tissue to these extraordinary sites.

NOSOCOMIAL INFECTION
(Accidental Implantation)

In all probability, *nosocomial* will be a new term in the lay person's vocabulary. Doctors usually use the word among themselves. They might be standing around the patient's bed examining a scar that does not seem to be healing properly. One doctor may comment, "It looks like a nosocomial infection to me." Translation: the patient did not have this infection before she was admitted to the hospital, but through negligence she has it now.

Let us return to an extension of the dandelion metaphor. An entire field of dandelions may yield a delightful bottle of dandelion wine. The enthusiast takes up garden shears and cuts the flowers to make the wine. One of the seeds catches in the scissor blades and later falls to the ground. The gardener has inadvertently sown the seed, and a dandelion becomes an unwanted weed.

A similar situation may be true in surgery involving the endometrial lining of the uterus. The prolific uterine lining provides a perfect home for a fetus. If the surgeon inadvertently transfers some of the uterine tissue while performing a Caesarian section or any other surgical procedure related to the uterus, however, the patient may end up with endometriosis as well as a baby, compliments of the surgeon.

These cases are not as rare as the medical profession would lead one to believe. They have been well documented in medical literature. Endometriosis has been found in women with no previous history of the condition, in whom it is usually discovered subsequent to surgery or diagnostic procedures related to the uterus.

Experiments have been conducted on laboratory animals in which endometrial tissue was deliberately transplanted into surgical scars. The implanted endometrial cells grew. Endometrial tissue is obviously quite viable, no matter what part of the body it inhabits or how it got there.

A recent article in the journal *Human Pathology* discusses endometriosis in surgical scars. The author observes, "The endometrial tissue grows along the line of penetration of the tissue by a suture."

A great percentage of the many cases of nosocomial infection involve obstetrical procedures. A woman can "catch" endometriosis if her doctor was not meticulous or careful enough in his or her examination or surgical technique. Some of the reported cases of the spread of endometriosis by surgery include laparotomy, episiotomy, Caesarian section, and, in some instances, even amniocentesis.

In these cases of endometriosis, the pregnant woman is not immune. In fact, she is vulnerable. The theory of accidental implantation proves an exception to the rule that pregnancy can curtail or even prevent endometriosis. To the contrary, pregnancy may lead to the introduction of endometriosis into the woman's system because of certain routine surgical procedures.

Many books have been written about the abnormal process of having babies in this country. Two of the most lucid include *Mal(e)practice: How Doctors Manipulate Women* by Robert Mendelsohn, M.D., and *A Woman in Residence* by Michelle Harrison, M.D. Both authors deplore the routine episiotomies (surgical enlargement of the vaginal opening) that are often performed on pregnant women, leaving painful scarring in the vaginal introitus area. Some women say that the episiotomy is more painful than having a baby. Walking can be difficult for several days because of tenderness and pain. Several months or even a year or so later, implants of endometriosis can become established around the scar. With the added complication of endometriosis just when the baby needs its mother, everyone suffers. The discovery of endometriosis in episiotomy and Caesarian scars might be reason enough to rethink routine obstetrical procedures currently practiced in a large number of hospitals across the United States.

INVASION OF THE UTERUS
(Adenomyosis)

A great number of researchers and doctors in the past have separated endometriosis and adenomyosis into two distinct categories, since the latter takes place in the uterus itself. *Aden* is Greek for gland, *mys* for muscle, and *osis* means an abnormal condition. Adenomyosis, then, is an abnormal glandular condition arising in the inner muscular wall of the uterus. An *adenomyoma* consists of a benign endometrial tumor composed of muscle and possessing glandular properties. Islands of misplaced endometrium are found in the smooth muscle. Another term for the condition is *endometriosis interna*, or internal endometriosis.

Usually, the mass very much resembles fibroid tumors, and like fibroids, it enlarges the uterus so that it appears swollen. Also like fibroids, the condition mostly affects older women nearing menopause.

If adenomyosis works from within the uterus, penetrating the inner muscular wall, is it not altogether different from endometriosis?

Womancare, a handbook for women's health, notes, "It is now thought that the two conditions are separate and distinct, so the term 'internal endometriosis' is no longer used."

Gynecologist Dr. Paul Manganiello of the Dartmouth-Hitchcock Medical Center says, "They're two different things, but basically the same process of ectopic endometrial tissue."

During a round-table discussion on endometriosis sponsored by the journal *Patient Care* and later recorded in that publication, Dr. Jaroslav Marik, Clinical Assistant Professor of Obstetrics and Gynecology at the University of California School of Medicine, comes to the same conclusion. When asked if adenomyosis is distinct from endometriosis, he replies, "They are the same disease."

To the contrary, in a monograph representing the contribution of several scholars meeting for a 1975 symposium on endometriosis, Dr. Abraham Rakoff pointed out, "Although adenomyosis is a form of endometriosis, it is in many ways a different disease in its clinical manifestations, pathologic characteristics, and management."

Two conflicting opinions about adenomyosis are being circulated by the medical profession. Are *endometriosis externa* and *endometriosis interna* one and the same condition arising in different locations? Or is endometriosis completely distinct from adenomyosis? This question should be answered, because as long as the confusion exists, some researchers will combine their statistics for both conditions and others will separate them, further complicating the research task. Consider two articles about the incidence of endometriosis in a black population in Nigeria. In one study, the researchers separated findings from endometriosis patients into those with adenomyosis and those with both conditions. In a different paper on the incidence of endometriosis in families, the researchers used the general term *endometriosis*, making no distinction.

Until doctors agree whether they are talking about two different types of oranges, or, in fact, about oranges and pears, many of the statistics being accumulated in the field today will be invalid. It is like starting a race at two different locations to arrive at the same goal.

3

More a Condition Than a Disease

ACCORDING TO *Webster's Ninth New Collegiate Dictionary*, a disease is a condition that "impairs the performance of a vital function." With endometriosis, however, some women function normally and are never aware they have it. Even when a woman wants to become pregnant, fertility experts observe that often her Fallopian tubes appear patent (open) with no sign of impairment of the reproductive system.

So the question might be asked, "Is endometriosis in fact a disease?" It has been proven that some endometrial tissue makes its way outside the normal uterine cavity in all women. Yet medical articles and encyclopedic entries refer to "out-of-place tissue," "the right thing in the wrong place," "endometrium in ectopic situations," "abnormally placed endometrial cells."

Gynecologists observe that endometriosis is a common condition that only in the intermediate and later stages can impair normal bodily function. Thus far, we have explored the nature of the condition in regard to the endometrium of the uterus, which somehow becomes implanted outside the uterus. But suppose that other forces in a woman's body were to play a part in the development of endometriosis. Now, the key word would not be *abnormal* but *predisposition.* In medicine, the term *abnormal* is usually paired with disease, whereas *predisposition* indicates susceptibility to a certain set of circumstances or condition. Disease denotes a force from without, a pathogen that invades the body; predisposition includes built-in factors, such as receptivity and immunity, heredity, hormonal levels, and individual tolerances.

It is important to take a long look at the body's defense mechanisms. Perhaps they might solve the mystery of why some women are affected by endometriosis and others are not.

When asked if he was close to discovering why a predisposition existed in some women, specialist Dr. Robert Kistner answered, "No. That's up to the immunologists. There's not much interest. There should be, but there's not."

Whether endometriosis is called a disease or a condition, it still affects an estimated 15 percent of women of reproductive age in this country. And this estimate is on the rise. The time has come, if not to answer questions, at least to ask them.

ANTIBODIES (The Immunologic Theory)

The key-lock analogy is ideal for speaking of the body's immune system. Each organism, such as a virus, that invades the body is stamped with a unique key, called an antigen. At the same time, the body's immune system consists of a variety of locks, or antibodies. When the right key fits into the appropriate lock, the invader is immediately targeted for destruction by specialized cells. The number of potentially different antibodies in a person's system can total 18 billion.

Cancer cells are known to carry surface markers that identify them to the immune system. It is possible that endometrial cells might also be marked. Dr. George T. Schneider, Professor of Obstetrics and Gynecology at the Louisiana State University of Medicine in New Orleans, agrees that there "may be some immunologic resistance in patients who don't develop endometriosis." Dr. Schneider adds that immunologic studies in New Orleans point to "an autoimmune phenomenon as a possible causative factor in infertility associated with endometriosis."

An increasing number of diseases are being associated with surface cell antigens and immune responses, or more appropriately, lack of them. Among these are multiple sclerosis, certain forms of arthritis, and juvenile diabetes.

In cancer research, many scientists have come to believe that everyone produces mutant cells, a few of them cancerous, but because of our highly evolved immune systems, such cells can be identified and destroyed. In all probability, such a theory could apply to unwanted endometrial tissue as well. The similarities between the dissemination routes of cancer and benign endometriosis have been acknowledged by researchers for more than half a century.

Gynecologist John Weed and immunologist Pierre Arquembourg of the Ochsner Medical Institutions in New Orleans have been studying the possibility of an autoimmune response in connection with infertility and endometriosis for some time. They have asked two important questions in their research. Why is endometriosis frequently related to primary infertility (inability to conceive) when it may not be incapacitating or clinically extensive? And why is secondary infertility (after a woman has had a child) overcome when the endometriosis is removed?

They propose that the answer might very well be that endometriosis causes an autoimmune response (sensitization to a substance produced by one's own body) that leads to both primary and secondary infertility. Their research thus far indicates that endometriosis creates an "antigen" from the woman's own endometrial proteins. These are recognized by her own body as "foreign." Dr. Weed writes that thus far they have been unable to isolate the "antigen." If they do, their discovery could unravel the mystery of infertility caused by endometriosis.

HORMONE LEVELS (Hormonal Imbalance)

At this juncture in gynecological research, we are gathering completely new and very exciting knowledge about the reproductive system. For example, we now know for certain that the hypothalamus and pituitary gland act as the control center for the ovaries. The hypothalamus is a part of the brain that lies just above a small oval endocrine gland, the pituitary. The brain relays a message to this gland to produce two hormones, follicle-stimulating hormone (FSH) and lutinizing hormone (LH).

FSH develops the ovum-containing follicles (sacs). As the ovaries and follicles develop, three types of estrogen are produced. In turn, these hormones prepare the uterine lining for the egg. A woman has a total of about four hundred eggs that will ripen in her lifetime (from a reserve of approximately half a million).

LH is transmitted by the pituitary gland to the ovaries. This hormone triggers the release of the egg from its follicle sac in the ovary.

In 1957 a British physiologist isolated other hormonelike substances from the menstrual tissue. These were prostaglandins that were found to stimulate the contraction of smooth muscles in the uterus. Fourteen prostaglandins to date have been identified in the human body. They exist in virtually every cell. In this case, however, the prostaglandins were discovered in the uterus. A correlation has been made between menstrual cramping and their presence in large amounts.

The reproductive drama, then, centers around hormones. Lead roles are played by estrogen, progesterone, and the prostaglandins, which advance and recede depending on the stage of a woman's menstrual cycle.

The final run occurs when the managing director, the pituitary, walks onstage and with heroic effort convinces producers FSH and LH to keep the show going. The increased production (by twenty times) causes total bankruptcy and subsequent hot flashes. Meanwhile, estrogen takes a bow in the ovaries.

What part endometriosis plays in this scenario, if any, is still not clear. A few doctors believe that hormonal imbalance could be a contributing factor. It has been proven, for example, that women with severe menstrual cramps produce more prostaglandins. In this connection one might note that the most common symptom of endometriosis is menstrual pain. It is also thought that prostaglandins dilate the blood vessels of the uterine lining, causing the release of excessive menstrual fluid—another symptom frequently found in endometriosis.

Results of prostaglandin studies indicate a significant elevation of prostaglandin levels in endometriosis patients. Preliminary findings tend to support a link between the manufacture of excess prostaglandins and the predisposition or hypersensitivity of some women to endometrial fragments.

During the 1950s, researchers discovered that the production of prostaglandins in the body could be inhibited by certain drugs. Most of these drugs were anti-inflammatory agents used for arthritis. Aspirin is a mild prostaglandin inhibitor. Today, prostaglandin inhibitors such as Motrin are prescribed to relieve menstrual cramps.

Do these same drugs inhibit endometriosis? A doctor may prescribe a prostaglandin inhibitor in an infertile patient in whom endometriosis is suspected. The inhibitor may relieve symptoms from mild endometriosis, but will not cause a severe case to recede. The use of prostaglandin inhibitors to treat endometriosis is still in the test stage.

THE BENIGN CANCER (Transformation)

The sobriquet "benign cancer" has been used by researchers in reference to endometriosis. In fact, Sampson's early publications conclude, "The invasion and dissemination of benign endometrial tissue employ the same channels as the invasion of cancer."

Those channels are: by invasion of neighboring tissue (benign adenomyosis invades the muscle wall of the uterine cavity); by getting into the blood or lymph system (this is the same explanation for how benign endometrial tissue reaches the underarm lymph nodes and other sites); by metastasis (after being transplanted, benign endometrial tissue grows—metastasizes—into a cyst or clump of implants).

As noted, some cancer specialists believe that we produce mutant cells, some of which may be cancer cells, but that our immune systems take care of destroying them. In part, this theory has been applied to explain endometriosis. Few researchers, however, accept the idea that undifferentiated cells mutate and thus form endometrial cells. They prefer the theory that the cells definitely originate in the uterus, after which the body's autoimmune response takes over.

Several correlations may be made between benign endometriosis and cancer. Women without children are vulnerable to endometrial cancer, and, it is said, also more vulnerable to endometriosis. According to *Womancare* on women's health, "Eighty percent of women with endometrial cancer have a history of menstrual irregularities." Women with endometriosis present similar histories.

But here the parallels stop. About half the women with forms of uterine cancer are overweight, whereas endometriosis has been associated with a trim, athletic body build. In endometrial cancer, inherited characteristics affect 12 to 20 percent of the patients, whereas for endometriosis (although studies are preliminary), only about 7 percent are so affected.

Endometriosis differs from cancer in at least three important respects. First, endometriosis does not digest the tissues of its host. It implants itself on the host but does not destroy tissue. Endometriosis is like a barnacle that glues itself onto a shell. At high tide (the menses) it becomes active, and at low tide it remains inactive.

Second, endometriosis has a much slower growth pattern than cancer. A woman may have endometriosis for fifteen years and not even be aware of the condition unless she tries to have children. In contrast, some breast and uterine cancers spread and grow at a fast pace.

Third, all endometriosis depends on ovarian function, whether it is found in the elbow or near the uterus. As one doctor said, "It has no mind of its own." Uterine and breast cancers depend on estrogen, but at least a hundred types of cancers exist and are caused by a variety of factors, including viruses and radiation.

Although it travels in the same channels as cancer, endometriosis takes orders from the ovaries and is dependent on estrogen. It rarely appears in males. Only three or four cases have been documented, and these were older men on *estrogen* therapy for prostate surgery.

Benign comes from the Latin word meaning kind. Endometriosis sufferers might object to calling endometriosis kind. The condition is rarely fatal, however, and perhaps that is the greatest difference of all between endometriosis and cancer.

FAMILY CONNECTIONS
(Genetic Predisposition)

Until 1980 no formal genetic studies on endometriosis had been published, so very little was known about whether the condition tended to run in families. At that time, four doctors collaborated on a study of 123 patients. All the patients had been diagnosed by laparotomy or laparoscopy with proven visualized endometriosis.

Nearly 6 percent of the patients' sisters were affected, and 8 percent of their mothers. One patient's mother and sister were both affected. Of two sets of twins (monozygotic or identical twins from one egg), both twins of one set had endometriosis, and in the other set, only one woman was affected. Data from distant relatives could not be relied on and so was excluded from the study.

Altogether, the likelihood that a first-degree relative (sister or mother) would have endometriosis turned out to be approximately 7 percent. The doctors emphasized in their report, however, that this figure in all probability represented an interaction between genetic and environmental factors. In genetics they call this "multifactorial inheritance."

One clue that led to their premise that endometriosis is probably a combination of family, environmental, and genetic influences came from the sets of twins. If endometriosis were entirely genetic, all identical twins would have it, but this was true for only three twins from two sets.

What did strike the doctors in their unique and important study was that *severe* cases of endometriosis showed a stronger genetic relationship. In fact, correlations showed that severe endometriosis involved 62 percent of the familial cases and only 23 percent of nonfamilial cases. This discovery underlines the necessity for doctors to pay close attention to taking family medical histories. If a patient's mother or sister had *severe* endometriosis, she has a much greater risk of developing the condition.

In high-risk cases, counseling could help the adolescent to make decisions about childbearing and contraceptive measures. For example, it has been observed that intrauterine devices cause endometriosis to proliferate. If the doctor finds a family history of endometriosis, she or he might suggest that the patient consider a progestin-dominant, low-estrogen oral contraceptive. Also, if the young patient with a known family history of severe endometriosis comes to the doctor with menstrual cramps, the doctor might advise an early pelvic exam and possible laparoscopy. Early detection and therapy could prevent more serious problems later.

Until more studies have been conducted, we must settle for 7 percent multifactorial family connections. For the present, factors such as a family tendency to late childbearing, inherent body build, and a difference in the genetically determined immune system might contribute in part or as a whole to endometriosis in families.

4

Symptoms

IMAGINE THAT A MOSQUITO flits through the room on a summer night. The mosquito is notorious for attacking the warmest and dampest parts of the body. It may land on the temple or on a vein in the neck, filling up on blood coursing through a tributary close to the skin. But if it misses its mark, the consequent lump and itching are not so bothersome. Bites near the eye or on the jugular vein will flare up and swell more than those on less vulnerable locations.

The same is true with endometriosis and its symptoms. Implants near nerve endings or conflicting directly with the functioning of certain organs are more likely to produce symptoms. An endometrial clump near the sciatic nerve will probably cause back pain, but many implants on the exterior wall of the uterus might not produce any symptoms at all.

Asymptomatic endometriosis affects an estimated 25 to 30 percent of endometriosis cases. What is without symptoms and harmless one day, however, may someday grow into a "gluestick disease," binding the organs and eventually producing overwhelming damage.

COMMON COMPLAINTS

Dysmenorrhea

Dysmenorrhea is the most frequent symptom associated with endometriosis. Dysmenorrhea means difficult and painful menstrual flow. When doctors speak of primary dysmenorrhea, they are referring to pelvic pain (usually in teenagers) where there seems to be no apparent organic cause.

In her book *Freedom from Menstrual Cramps*, Dr. Kathryn Schrotenboer of New York City notes that smaller masses of endometriosis often seem to cause more pain than larger ones. Authority Dr. Robert Kistner of the Harvard Medical School has observed large cysts on the ovaries with extensive adhesions that produced no pain. He reflects, "This absence of pain must be accounted for by something more than individual differences in pain threshold and may be due to the exceedingly slow rate of distention of the endometrial cysts."

How long does the pain last? A few health books state that pain is experienced only during the woman's period, while others indicate that the pain may start two or three weeks prior to and continue during menstruation. A recent article on endometriosis in *Mademoiselle* asserts, "The characteristic which distinguishes these symptoms from common menstrual cramps is the recent onset of symptoms, of a pattern of symptoms where none had been present before."

Of women interviewed for this book, however, several mentioned a long and complicated history of menstrual pain and distress. One endometriosis sufferer from Massachusetts said that she had a heavy flow from the onset of her periods. Another woman from Washington, D.C., remembered always having cramps with her periods.

One of the first questions a doctor asks is, "What kind of pain do you have?" We all know how difficult it is to describe pain. Even at the dentist it seems impossible to point to the tooth causing the toothache. We would like to assume that is the doctor's job.

Although we wish doctors were mind readers, they are not. A precise description of symptoms may provide the doctor with clues so that he or she may be able to make a diagnosis. It is your body, and you are best qualified to explain how you feel. The doctor might help by suggesting, "Is the pain sharp and jabbing? Dull? Throbbing? A twinge or an ache? Localized or dispersed?"

Be ready as a patient to define "painful periods" with definite, well-thought-out information.

- When does the pain start? Before, during, after the menstrual period? Keep monthly records.
- What is the pain like?
- Where is it located?
- Has the pain worsened progressively? Have you always had menstrual cramps?
- How does the pain affect your life-style? Is the pain disabling?

In his foreword to papers evolving from a conference on endometriosis, Dr. Robert Greenblatt, Professor Emeritus of Endocrinology at the Medical College of Georgia, advises that "every young woman with dysmenorrhea should be suspect [of endometriosis]."

Unfortunately, some doctors tend to regard patients with complaints of chronic menstrual pain as nervous, under stress, and in need of a psychologist. A discussion among endometriosis specialists recorded in *Patient Care* describes what could happen.

Dr. B.: Do you often encounter patients with significant endometriosis who've been dismissed by their referring physicians as chronic pain "crocks"?

Dr. S.: It happens frequently.

Dr. M.: It's especially likely to happen if the woman says, "My mother had pain and my sister has pain." It's very easy to assume a psychological overlay, especially if you [the doctor] aren't attuned to the frequency of endometriosis today.

The responsibility, then, must be assumed by the patient. If she knows what endometriosis is and has analyzed to the best of her ability how, when, and where the pain occurs, it will be difficult to dismiss her with a bottle of painkillers or refer her to the nearest "shrink."

Dyspareunia

Dyspareunia means difficult or painful intercourse and represents another common symptom of endometriosis. Sex may be painful because of lesions and endometrial implants in an area called the cul-de-sac or pouch of Douglas. This pouch is a sort of dead end between the back of the uterine wall and the rectum. Endometrial tissue frequently is trapped in this area, causing a freezing or fixation of the uterus in a retroverted position.

Any form of deep vaginal penetration with the uterus locked into this position can cause a sharp jabbing pain. Such pain may be a contributing factor to another symptom of endometriosis, namely, infertility. Because of associated pain, the endometriosis sufferer might ask her sexual partner to ease off or avoid intercourse completely, thus reducing the chances for pregnancy.

Backache

Endometriosis in the cul-de-sac may also produce lower backache during the menstrual period. According to specialist Dr. Robert Kistner, "Every ectopic endometrial gland is a miniature uterine cavity that can menstruate coincidentally with the uterus and produce blood for which there is no avenue of escape."

The pain from this engorgement of blood radiates out and into the lower back. Most humans standing on two feet complain of lower back pain at some time in their lives. When the pain arrives during a woman's menstrual period, however, she should consider endometriosis.

Painful Defecation and Rectal Bleeding

Constipation, rectal bleeding, and painful defecation during the menstrual period can all point to endometriosis. Blockage of the bowel and implants in the rectal area will bring on these symptoms.

Common hemorrhoids, however, may elicit similar complaints. Careful attention should be paid to the appearance of these symptoms in conjunction with the menstrual period. Any bleeding from the rectum should, of course, immediately be reported to the doctor.

Infertility

An estimated 25 to 40 percent of all women with an infertility problem have endometriosis. As yet, doctors have not discovered exactly why. Often, the endometrial implants are small and relatively few. Also, in most patients the Fallopian tubes seem patent (open) and functional.

Infertility is the endometriosis symptom most gynecologists recognize and subsequently treat. A majority of current research studies being done on endometriosis relate to infertility. A number of gynecologists drawn to the field are interested in what one physician referred to as "the baby-making business." For women who desperately want families, the known connection between endometriosis and infertility provides an inbuilt system for reliable diagnosis and consequent treatment. But for women who are not focused on fertility, women with symptoms of pain and irregular menses, the road to diagnosis and treatment can be long and erratic.

Menstrual Irregularities

Excessive flow (menorrhagia) and spot bleeding (metorrhagia) are more commonly associated with cases of *endometriosis interna,* a condition of endometrial invasion of the uterine wall in older women (see pp. 130–31).

But menstrual irregularities may also be symptoms of *endometriosis externa.* Symptoms vary from woman to woman and may be related to a number of factors, including age. The entire complex of symptoms always arises in relation to the woman's individual menstrual cycle. Any irregularities in that cycle, including excessive flow and premenstrual spotting, should be checked out by a gynecologist, especially when the symptoms persist or worsen.

One woman from New Hampshire relates, "For as long as I could remember I had heavy and painful periods. There was so little information in those days that one didn't know if this was normal or not. The other thing that concerned me was blood clots. They were always extremely hard to explain to physicians. There would be instances where I would be with colleagues in meetings and be afraid to stand up."

The idea has been perpetuated that most adolescents suffer from some sort of menstrual irregularity at the onset. But recent studies on endometriosis in teenagers are leading to a heightened awareness that more attention should be paid to early complaints of heavy and painful periods in young women.

Other Symptoms

Each symptom that appears might give a clue to the location of endometrial implants. Implants on the sheath of the sciatic nerve, for example, can cause pain radiating from the buttocks to the thigh and along the outside of the leg. One woman in Boston remembered, "The pain radiated down into my legs most of the time, not just during menstruation."

A SYMPTOM SAMPLER

J.K., a teacher and an artist now working in Montana and mother of one son, recognized her symptoms and immediately connected them with endometriosis. Unfortunately, the gynecologists did not. They told her this was just the way she was, although her mother and grandmother both had had hysterectomies, and her mother's hysterectomy was performed because of severe endometriosis and fibroids.

All the symptoms experienced by J.K. are more readily associated with endometriosis today. In order for the reader to form a better picture of a vivid and pronounced set of endometriosis symptoms, here is J.K.'s account.

I had my first period when I was fifteen. My periods lasted seven-and-a-half days. My mother had her hysterectomy the day I started my period, which was sort of a family joke because I'd be carrying on the fertility of the family at the time she was having hers terminated. I would go through twenty-four sanitary napkins. I'd double them. I always passed clots and I also had lower backaches.

At nineteen I had my first hemorrhage. Before, I'd had dreadful pain in my right side and missed my period. I've never had such pain, including childbirth. There was spotting between my periods, too.

I was hospitalized and given my first D&C [dilation and curettage, or surgical scraping of the uterine wall]. For a year and a half I didn't spot. Then I started breakthrough bleeding. So I went to another doctor. I was married at twenty-three and they put me on the Pill, but I vomited continually so I quit after three months. Then I got pregnant and had an easy pregnancy. I started breakthrough bleeding again.

When I was in my early thirties the pain returned to my right side so that I was buckled over most of the time. Finally, I went to a specialist. He told me I had endometriosis, and I had a hysterectomy. The endometriosis had spread everywhere. It was all over the appendix. The right ovary was covered. My whole rectum was totally full.

From the first pain at fifteen until before my hysterectomy in my early thirties, I believed I was suffering from endometriosis. So many doctors didn't believe me, but I knew myself.

Although less easy to distinguish on one's own, anemia often accompanies endometriosis because of heavy periods, loss of iron in the blood through extensive endometrial implants, and energy expended because of associated pain.

COMMON SITES FOR ENDOMETRIOSIS

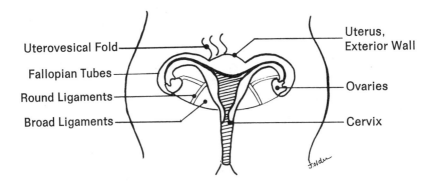

Uterovesical Fold
Fallopian Tubes
Round Ligaments
Broad Ligaments

Uterus, Exterior Wall
Ovaries
Cervix

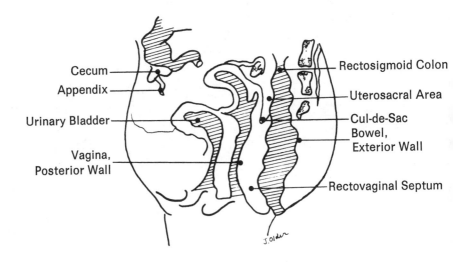

Cecum
Appendix
Urinary Bladder
Vagina, Posterior Wall

Rectosigmoid Colon
Uterosacral Area
Cul-de-Sac
Bowel, Exterior Wall
Rectovaginal Septum

LESS COMMON SITES FOR ENDOMETRIOSIS

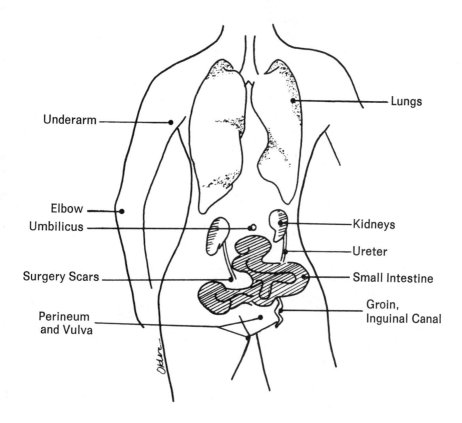

A woman with endometriosis does not run a temperature, but her white cell count may be high. This, in connection with manifest pain and menstrual distress, may be ample evidence for the discerning gynecologist to recommend laparoscopy.

SYMPTOMS AND SITES

Symptoms	*Probable Area of Endometriosis*
Painful intercourse	Vagina, Cul-de-sac
Rectal bleeding, painful defecation (especially during menstruation), constipation	Bowel wall
Infertility, premenstrual staining	Ovaries and Fallopian tubes
Dyspareunia, heavy bleeding during periods	Cul-de-sac with retroverted uterus, fixed uterus
Urinary frequency, pus in the urine, urinary retention, pain in the flank and groin, blood in the urine during menstruation	Bladder and urethra
Vomiting, abdominal pain, abdominal swelling	Small intestine
Bulges tender and painful to the touch, especially as menstruation approaches	Umbilicus, thighs, forearms, lungs
Pain radiating from buttocks to the outside legs	Sciatic nerve
Flank pain on the affected side	Kidney (rare)
Symptoms similar to acute appendicitis; pain before menstruation	Appendix
Coughing of blood during menstruation; pneumonialike symptoms with fever as it spreads	Thorax, lungs

CHOOSING A DOCTOR

In came the doctor, in came the nurse
In came the lady with a notebook in her purse.

Up to a certain point, we may speculate on our own symptoms, but after careful observation and recording, we must relate this information to a physician. Whom do we see? The gynecologist? The family doctor? An endometriosis specialist? A surgeon? Planned Parenthood? The neighborhood clinic? Mother? The main criterion is to select someone who will *listen*.

Actually, talking with one's mother or sister is a good idea because their gynecological and menstrual problems might lead to a better understanding of your own, and might provide a medical background for the physician.

Keep in mind that diagnosing endometriosis involves many steps, and your first visit is just to deal with the preliminaries. Not all gynecologists will recognize endometriosis, nor will all family practitioners, nor the registered nurse at a health clinic. But they should be able to refer the woman who thinks she has endometriosis to a specialist. They can also make preliminary blood tests and perform a pelvic exam to feel for endometrial masses and nodules.

This initial visit will probably start with the question, "Well now, what's bothering you today?" A word to the wise. Do not jump to conclusions. Remember, the diagnosis depends on what the doctor finds. So describe your symptoms and give the doctor time to form an opinion.

It is advisable to write down dates of menstrual cycles and accompanying symptoms in a notebook. If asked, you may bring up family-related problems. You should try not to be emotional about pain. Just the facts. No embroidery. The truth may be that last month you felt as if you were going to die, but the doctor only wants to know where, when, and how long. Today's practitioners often have only half an hour or less to take a medical history and examine each patient.

Find out what tests are being done and why. Ask for a urinalysis and a blood count. If the doctor finds nothing extraordinary during the exam and has not suggested a follow-up exam *during* the next menstrual period, perhaps the next step may be to consult an endometriosis specialist. The best time to have a complete pelvic exam is the day before or during your period, because at this time the implants are swollen with blood, making them more likely to be discovered. Also, lab work at this time may show blood in the urine or feces.

If a patient does have endometriosis, however, and is given a rough pelvic exam by a brusque, hurried gynecologist who pumps and prods unnecessarily, the endometrial implants could spread, especially during menstruation. So perhaps the wisest procedure would be first to visit the hometown gynecologist or family clinic while you are not menstruating. If you still suspect endometriosis, but the exam reveals no evidence, you may contact a specialist. More than likely, the specialist will want to do still another pelvic exam, and then if endometriosis is suspected, repeat the exam during the menstrual period. Most endometriosis specialists are aware that careful and meticulous examination and diagnostic procedures are crucial to the containment of endometrial implants.

When asked what to advise women who think they might have the condition, one ex-patient replied, "I would definitely go to a specialist who works with endometriosis, or to a good larger hospital with a qualified staff. At least provide yourself with *three* different opinions." Another woman responded, "It's very important to look for a good doctor, and if the endometriosis is bad, a good surgeon."

A newspaper reporter pressed by debilitating pain went to a gynecologist and after a pelvic exam was told she had endometriosis. Terrified that she had some form of cancer, she asked for an explanation. The doctor shoved a medical text into her lap and went off to use the phone. Such behavior is not the norm. You should, however, be psychologically prepared for two or three visits to different doctors.

Perhaps the best advice comes from a New England college teacher who passed through several hospital corridors on her way to a correct diagnosis. "A friend of mine has endometriosis and is going to have conservative surgery. I told her, 'Listen, you don't have to sit there without your clothes on and talk to him. Just say you want to talk to him in detail when it's convenient for both of you and he'll do it.' "

A "talking" appointment is the time to lay the cards on the table. Be informed. Ask questions. Do not be reticent simply because the doctor knows more than you do about the condition. The physician has the knowledge, but you have the endometriosis. We all are entitled to results of biopsies, laboratory reports, information pertaining to physical examinations, and, most important, to common courtesy.

DISEASES WITH SIMILAR SYMPTOMS

It should be understood that the diagnosis of endometriosis may be complicated by several other diseases presenting quite similar symptoms. This phenomenon happens in nature a great deal. For example, many snakes look like the poisonous coral snake at first glance, but unless their bands follow the red, yellow, black, yellow order, they're not. At first glance, endometriosis may often appear to be something else. The following conditions can obscure correct diagnosis.

PID (Pelvic Inflammatory Disease)

PID seems to be the disease four out of five doctors suggest when the patient complains of lower back pain, painful intercourse, cramps, difficult defecation, spot bleeding, tenderness, and a host of other symptoms. PID is an infection caused by bacteria and can be cleared up by antibiotics.

Women who suspect that they have endometriosis might

have to submit to antibiotic treatment just to rule out the possibility of PID. If antibiotics fail to relieve the symptoms, however, the search should continue for the underlying problem.

A few other differences help the doctor to distinguish between PID and endometriosis. During the pelvic exam, PID will sometimes show masses of infection that are tender and fluctuate. But in endometriosis, the masses usually are quite firm.

Also, if a Rubin test (an office procedure in which carbon dioxide is passed through the Fallopian tubes) is performed and the tubes are found to be blocked, more than likely the diagnosis will be PID, not endometriosis. Unfortunately, this is the test of preference performed on women who want to become pregnant, and it is rarely prescribed otherwise.

It is interesting to interject that until recently (and no doubt even now, by some doctors who should know better) PID was equated with black women and endometriosis with white women. This sort of mental triage was primarily based on the dichotomy between the black ward patient and the more affluent white private patient. The facts have established that endometriosis exists in both black and white women, a topic discussed at length in chapter 14.

Appendicitis

Often, a woman with severe pain in her right side is thought to have appendicitis. When a large ovarian cyst is about to rupture, however, it can cause symptoms very much like acute appendicitis.

It is not uncommon for the surgeon to rush the patient to the operating room and find the appendix adhered to other organs in a weblike adhesion of endometrial tissue. The surgeon might also find an ovarian cyst about to rupture, rather than an infected appendix.

Involvement of endometriosis with the appendix is common; in fact, many surgeons recommend removal of the appendix while operating on other areas of endometriosis, even though the appendix is not yet affected. Dr. Kistner says, "I never do anything routinely, but since the appendix is involved by the endometriotic process in approximately 8 to 9 percent of cases, particularly in its later stages, I will usually remove it."

Ectopic Pregnancy

Endometriosis adhering to the tubes may be misdiagnosed as ectopic pregnancy. Dr. L. Iffy, a researcher who has extensively studied ectopic pregnancies, reports in the *International Journal of Fertility* that the egg of an ectopic pregnancy is fertilized late in the woman's menstrual cycle, too late to prevent the next menstrual period. He speculates that when the woman menstruates, pieces of endometrial tissue travel with the fertilized egg into the Fallopian tubes, instead of exiting through the cervix. His research thus far demonstrates that the embryo from an ectopic pregnancy is usually one month more developed than the woman's menstrual history would indicate. So when ectopic pregnancy is diagnosed, there might be a close connection with ectopic endometrial tissue as well.

Apart from this important discovery, ectopic pregnancy does produce symptoms of pain in the abdominal region that could also resemble those of an ovarian endometrial cyst or extensive endometriosis elsewhere in the pelvic region.

Diverticulitis

Diverticulitis is an inflammation of the diverticula, or pouches that line the intestines in some people. The condition mostly affects older men and women. It can be congenital or acquired, but the symptoms are abdominal pain, constipation, and sometimes fever. Treatment includes dietary restriction and a cycle of tetracycline. Like PID, if the recommended treatment does not work, the woman should consider consulting a gynecologist specializing in endometriosis, especially if symptoms seem aggravated during menstruation.

Hernia

Endometriosis of the groin can often be mistaken as a hernia (an abnormal protrusion of an abdominal organ through a gap into the inguinal canal of the groin). If the tenderness in the groin becomes unbearable during the menstrual period, however, endometriosis should be suspected.

Cancer

If the doctor suspects cancer, chances are that the diagnostic procedure will be fast and thorough in order to eliminate any doubt. As already mentioned, endometriosis has been given the misnomer "benign cancer" more than once.

Endometriosis of the umbilicus, more commonly known as the navel or belly button, is often associated with metastatic cancer until a biopsy is performed. Again, tenderness of that area directly connected with menstruation can help to confirm the biopsy report for endometriosis.

An ovarian endometrial cyst and ovarian cancer are difficult to tell apart except through biopsy and laparoscopy. They both produce pelvic pain, although with ovarian cancer the woman usually loses weight, feels weak, and is noticeably anemic.

Some cancers of the rectum are known to implant and build a "rectal shelf," which may result in backache, constipation, and bleeding from the rectum—all symptoms of extensive endometriosis. Whenever these symptoms appear, they should be checked without delay.

Nodules

Many conditions of the body form nodular masses. As explained earlier, adenomyosis (*endometriosis interna*) is considered the same as endometriosis by some professionals and as an entirely different condition by others. The pelvic region of the adenomyosis patient can be tender with nodular masses. *Endometriosis externa* occurs in conjunction with *endometriosis interna* in about 20 percent of cases. The difference is that the common symptom of *endometriosis interna* is heavy bleeding in 85 percent of the women (with pain in 30 percent of cases). Also, the uterus of the adenomyosis patient is frequently enlarged.

Oxyuris vermicularis (threadworms) can cause calciferous nodules in the cul-de-sac, an area associated with endometriosis.

Another disease presents nodular lesions in the Fallopian tubes. It is called *salpingitis isthmica nodosa* and often shows up in the older patient undergoing a workup for infertility. This condition usually is not connected with symptoms of pelvic pain.

In ovarian cancer the nodules of the cul-de-sac are solid and resemble endometriosis very closely.

Cysts

Ovarian cysts are of several kinds, with various characteristics. Two types are follicle and corpus luteum cysts. Dr. Abraham Rakoff, in a paper titled "Differential Diagnosis Between Endometriosis and Other Conditions Causing Pelvic Pain and Dysmenorrhea," states that the "bleeding into a follicle or corpus luteum cyst can produce the same picture [as endometriosis]."

An endometrial cyst is called an endometrioma, and it differs from some other cysts in a few respects. For example, Dr. Rakoff explains that there is rarely a twisting in the endometrioma because by the time it is large enough to do so, it has already adhered firmly to the ovary.

With cysts, as with other problems of this nature, direct visualization by laparoscopy and biopsy are the only reliable diagnostic procedures.

Gonorrhea

A woman presenting symptoms of postmenstrual tenderness, discharge, and pelvic pain aggravated by intercourse might be given a smear or a culture for gonorrhea.

Advanced gonorrhea can lead to tubo-ovarian abscesses that spread and release pus into the pelvic cavity, causing widespread inflammation. If left untreated, the symptoms closely resemble endometriosis with abnormal bleeding, dysmenorrhea, and pelvic pain. Frequently, however, fever and chills accompany the symptom pattern and should give a clue that endometriosis probably is not involved. Antibiotics are the prescribed method of treatment. If there has been misdiagnosis, the antibiotic course will not be effective, and endometriosis should be considered.

The job of the physician in distinguishing endometriosis from other diseases is not always easy. With the cooperation of a well-informed, observant patient who has recorded her symptoms, however, the physician may formulate a logical method to narrow down the possibilities.

5

Infertility:
A Major Symptom

CONSERVATIVE ESTIMATES point to endometriosis as the cause of 30 percent of infertility in women, and some doctors believe it is closer to 40 percent.

THE INFERTILITY WORKUP

For the couple that desires children, the realization that they are infertile can come as a terrible shock. Popular women's magazines frequently print stories by women who have been unable to conceive, describing their consequent odyssey through infertility clinics. Sometimes they succeed in becoming pregnant and carrying the child to term. Others must adopt children. Often, the psychological threat of sterility separates the couple or leads to divorce.

The infertility clinic can often be a cold, matter-of-fact place where the doctor has heard the same story hundreds of times and may only be interested in the sperm count and how often the couple has sex. One infertile patient described her first visit: "They stood around me mumbling. One lifted my gown and pronounced, 'Nope, no hairs on her chest.' I was nearly in tears."

The infertility workup requires psychological and physical stamina. Some couples wait five years or more to start a family. Most important for the couple who cannot seem to become pregnant is to find a doctor who will listen to their problem and treat them as human beings.

Sex for a Year

Most infertility experts define infertility as the inability to become pregnant after a year of regular sexual activity. This definition usually does not count sexual activity prior to the appeal for help. Carol Pogash, at thirty, wanted to have a child. In a *Redbook* story, she recounts, "[My doctor said] that becoming pregnant was sometimes a year-long process, and recommended that my husband and I have intercourse every other day from the tenth through the twenty-second day of each cycle."

Sex by the calendar can be a strain on any couple and may turn a fulfilling sex life into a stressful situation. But a year of calendar sex without pregnancy seems to be the deciding factor indicating that a fertility problem exists.

Basal Temperature Charts

Before treatment for infertility is begun, it is essential to determine whether the woman is able to ovulate.

Doctors tend to disagree on whether or not recording a woman's temperature shows definite proof of ovulation. Dr. Jaroslav Marik, Professor of Obstetrics and Gynecology at the University of California School of Medicine, says, "To my mind the best evidence of ovulation is, first, of course, pregnancy; second, recovery of an egg from the tube or uterus; and third, visualization of the corpus luteum with stigma of ovulation on the surface of the ovary. After that, there's what I call *indirect* evidence: cervical mucous, vaginal cytology, hormone assays, and basal body temperature."

Carol Pogash's doctor believed that a rise in basal body temperature was proof of ovulation. In her article she relates, "Every morning, before moving so much as a toe from the bed, I slid a thermometer under my tongue." She recorded her temperature in this manner for nearly five years!

A basal thermometer is a special thermometer on which each degree is divided into very small fractions for accuracy. If the woman's temperature rises at midcycle (which varies from woman to woman), the theory is that she is ovulating. Sexual intercourse at this time should be optimum for conception, unless there is an infertility problem.

Some women with endometriosis can ovulate, but some cannot. In fact, one study showed that up to 40 percent of endometriosis patients were not ovulating. Nevertheless, such a woman can still have uterine bleeding.

One might assume that if more than a third of all infertile women have endometriosis, to chart the basal body temperature makes no sense. Precious time could be saved by trying to determine if the infertile woman has endometriosis in the first place, since endometriosis is a leading cause of infertility. One of the foremost endometriosis experts in the country emphasizes that the diagnosis of endometriosis should *always* be considered in infertile patients, especially if the leading symptoms are present.

Carol Pogash did have endometriosis, but three or four years passed before she found out about it.

Sperm Count

If the year of having sex by the calendar bears no results, next on the agenda is for the male partner to have a sperm count. Many factors—such as a high fever during childhood, sexually transmitted disease, undescended testicles, abnormalities in the testicles, and even heat from frequent hot tubs or athletic supporters—can slow down the sperm and cause a low sperm count.

Chronic illness, including addiction to drugs and alcohol or illnesses caused by toxic pesticides and environmental pollutants, such as PCBs, Agent Orange, and radiation, can also affect the sperm count. According to the gynecological handbook *Womancare*, "The average sperm count in American men has fallen by as much as 30% in the last 30 years." Much depends on sperm delivery (ejaculation) and the motility (movement) of the sperm. Sometimes hormones can be used to improve a low sperm count. If the problem is motility, the sperm may be saved and artificially inseminated into the partner. But if the count is in the normal spectrum, it is time for still other tests.

Postcoital Test

Another name for the postcoital test is the Huhner test. The woman must be at the doctor's office within a few hours after sexual intercourse without washing or douching. A sample of mucous from the cervix is obtained and examined under a microscope to determine if the partner's sperm have been able to get through the mucous and survive. The test is performed during the time a woman calculates that she is ovulating.

The consistency of cervical mucous differs at various points in the woman's reproductive cycle. She can learn to distinguish these various changes and eventually will be able to tell if she is ovulating. The greatest amount of mucous occurs at ovulation, changing from a scant thick substance to a thin clear fluid that permits the sperm to swim through. If the mucous is too thick at ovulation, the sperm may not be able to penetrate it.

Let us return to Carol Pogash's case. Years went by, and she commiserated with a cousin who had the same problem. Over the phone the cousin explained that her particular problem seemed to be endometriosis. She was taking hormones for it.

Had Pogash known about the familial incidence of endometriosis, she might have gone to her doctor and suggested that her infertility workup begin intensive testing for endometriosis.

Rubin Insufflation Test

The Rubin test is a simple office procedure that introduces carbon dioxide into the Fallopian tubes to see if they are blocked. With endometriosis, however, the tubes are rarely blocked. So this test is wonderful for showing other problems leading to infertility, but not endometriosis. The Rubin test produces mild shoulder pain because of the carbon dioxide in the system.

Hysterosalpingogram

Called a hysterogram by those who would rather not try pronouncing hysterosalpingogram, this test is a contrast x-ray taken after dye has been injected into the uterus. The test outlines the Fallopian tubes and uterus on a corresponding screen, showing any blockage. The dye disperses into the pelvic cavity with little discomfort.

Nearly all these tests are performed on women who want to become pregnant, and not necessarily for women with endometriosis who want to become pregnant. Most doctors agree that the only sure way to tell if a woman has endometriosis is by combined endoscopy (visualization of endometrial implants with a light-optic instrument) and biopsy.

By this time the patient, like Carol Pogash, may have gone through years of tests before the doctor decides to send her to the hospital for a laparoscopy. Ironically, by the time endometriosis is discovered and the woman has gone through six months of hormones and perhaps even conservative surgery, the odds against her conceiving when she is thirty-five years old, as opposed to twenty-nine or thirty, are much greater. Age definitely influences the chances for fertility in all women.

Women impatient to conceive, who think their symptoms have pointed to endometriosis all along and know they are not getting any younger, should press for diagnostic procedures that rule out endometriosis on their very first visit to the infertility specialist.

BEING CLASSIFIED

Until 1978 the most popular classification for endometriosis was into mild, moderate, and severe categories. Practitioners often differed, however, in their opinion of what constituted the various degrees of the condition. A definite classification was long ovedue. Finally, The American Fertility Society solicited a committee of endometriosis specialists to convene and establish a reliable system.

In use today, this classification is based on a simple point system to chart the progression of the disease. The doctor is encouraged to examine the pelvic area in a thorough clockwork fashion, indicating the number, size, and location of all endometriomas and implants.

For example, let us take five separate endometrial implants on the surface of the uterus. Let us say that each is 0.5 centimeters (2.5 cm total). According to the chart, a total area of 1 to 3 centimeters would be given 2 points. The points are added up, totaled, and categorized into four separate stages.

THE AMERICAN FERTILITY SOCIETY
STAGING TABLE

Stages of Endometriosis	*Points*
Stage I (mild)	1–5
Stage II (moderate)	6–15
Stage III (severe)	16–30
Stage IV	31–54

A sketch of the uterus, Fallopian tubes, and ovaries is provided on a blank patient worksheet. This worksheet resembles the dentist's record for cavities on which caries present in each tooth are indicated. On this drawing, the gynecologist may pinpoint where the endometriosis is located. The gynecologist then marks down where the endometriosis is located and how much area it covers, and checks the point score. The classification chart on the following page is referred to in order to determine the points. From this point system the gynecologist can then categorize the case as mild, moderate, or severe, according to the staging table above.

For example, if the patient has two filmy adhesions of 1 centimeter each on the peritoneum (2 points) and the right ovary has a dense adhesion of 3 centimeters (4 points), the gynecologist would record a total of 6 points. According to the staging table, she has "moderate endometriosis."

The illustration on pages 52–53 provides a picture of how endometriosis spreads and what areas are affected in the four stages.

Classification is made during laparoscopy or other diagnostic procedures in which the physician can visualize the endometriosis. Treatment should not be recommended until this classification is made.

If infertility is the problem, sperm tests, endometrial biopsy, tubal insufflation, and postcoital tests should be performed with laparoscopy within the year. If the woman does have stage III or IV endometriosis, time is of the essence. Her fertility is not only endangered, but she might have to face ultimate castration.

CHANCES OF FERTILITY

Figures vary in regard to the reversal rate for endometriosis patients who are infertile; the figures most often cited tend to

THE AMERICAN FERTILITY SOCIETY CLASSIFICATION

PERITONEUM

Endometriosis	1 cm	1–3 cm	3 cm
Points	1	2	3

Adhesions	filmy	dense w/ partial cul-de-sac obliteration	dense w/ complete cul-de-sac obliteration
Points	1	2	3

OVARY

Endometriosis	1 cm	1–3 cm	3 cm or ruptured endometrioma
Points R	2	4	6
Points L	2	4	6

Adhesions	filmy	dense w/ partial ovarian closure	dense w/ complete ovarian closure
Points R	2	4	6
Points L	2	4	6

FALLOPIAN TUBES

Endometriosis	1 cm	1 cm	tubal occlusion
Points R	2	4	6
Points L	2	4	6

Adhesions	filmy	dense w/ tubal distortion	dense w/ tubal enclosure
Points R	2	4	6
Points L	2	4	6

This chart is reproduced with permission of The American Fertility Society. Birmingham, Alabama.

CLASSIFICATION OF ENDOMETRIOSIS

STAGE I

Broad ligaments:
  No implants more than 5mm

Tubes:
  Avascular adhesions,
  fimbria free

Ovaries:
  Avascular adhesions,
  no fixation

Cul-de-sac: No implants more than 5mm

Bowel: Normal   Appendix: Normal

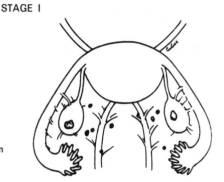

STAGE II, A

Broad ligaments:
  No implants more than 5 mm

Tubes:
  Avascular adhesions,
  fimbria free

Ovaries:
  Endometrial cyst 5cm or less,
  A1 stage; over 5cm, A2;
  ruptured, A3

Cul-de-sac: No implants more than 5mm

Bowel: Normal   Appendix: Normal

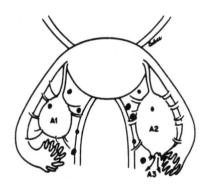

STAGE II, B

Broad ligaments:
  Covered by adherent ovary

Tubes:
  Adhesions not removable by endoscopy;
  fimbria free

Ovaries:
  Fixed to the broad ligament;
  implants over 5 mm

Cul-de-sac: Multiple implants,
  no adherent bowel or fixed uterus

Bowel: Normal   Appendix: Normal

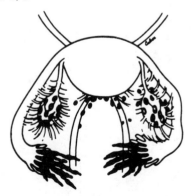

STAGE III

Broad ligaments:
  May be covered by adherent tube or ovary

Tubes: Fimbria are covered by adhesions

Ovaries:
  Adherent with or without
  implants or endometriomas

Cul-de-sac: Multiple implants,
  no adherent bowel or fixed uterus

Bowel: Normal   Appendix: Normal

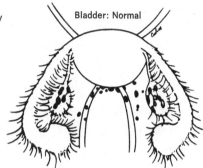

Bladder: Normal

STAGE IV
(Usually combined with stage I, II, III)

Bladder: Implants

Uterus: May be fixed and adherent posteriorly

Cul-de-sac: Covered by adherent bowel
  or fixed retrodisplaced uterus

Bowel: Adherent to the cul-de-sac,
  uterosacral ligaments, or corpus

Appendix: May be involved

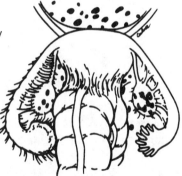

be from 25 to 40 percent. The chances for conception in women with mild endometriosis (stages I and II) naturally are much greater.

In two studies conducted by Harvard's Dr. Robert Kistner and colleagues, 76 percent of 232 women in stages I and II became pregnant after surgical treatment for endometriosis, whereas only 38 percent of 106 patients in stages III and IV responded to surgical treatment with subsequent pregnancies. The reversal rate also depends on the age of the woman. In his desk drawer Dr. Kistner keeps a chart to remind patients how age plays a dramatic part in a woman's fertility.

Age	Infertility
20–24	4.4%
25–29	5.4%
30–34	11%
35–39	20%

It has been shown that endometriosis can be fairly mild to moderate and still cause infertility. This phenomenon puzzles the researchers. For the most part, a lot of supposing has been done with little hard evidence as to why this happens.

Some doctors conjecture that infertility is the result of reduced sexual activity due to the pain that intercourse causes in some women with endometriosis. Another supposition focuses on the presence of a fixed, retroverted uterus and the displacement of the cervix, which could provide less accessibility for the sperm. If the sperm count is on the low side too, these two factors combined might make a difference.

Adhesions of endometriosis to the fimbrial ends of the Fallopian tubes (which guide the ovum into the tube) might inhibit their normal functioning.

Another guess is that endometriosis causes a dysfunction of the corpus luteum, the yellowish ovarian tissue formed from the ruptured follicle after it releases the ovum. It produces progesterone, which prepares the endometrium to receive the ovum. Abnormal function of the corpus luteum may lead to hormonal imbalance.

Prostaglandins

Take a good look at the word *prostaglandins*. We are going to be hearing much more about prostaglandins in the future.

Prostaglandins are hormone amino-acidlike substances that have been accused by some researchers of being responsible for menstrual cramps (primary dysmenorrhea). They are released prior to and during menstruation, causing the smooth muscles of the uterus to contract.

Women who suffer from menstrual cramping have been found to produce more prostaglandins. Researchers have found that prostaglandin inhibitors, drugs initially prescribed for arthritis, work effectively on most patients with severe dysmenorrhea. Drugs currently being prescribed for primary dysmenorrhea include naproxen sodium (Anaprox), ibuprofen (Motrin), fenoprofen calcium (Nalfon 200), and a medicine cabinet of others. The dosage usually prescribed is much less for a woman with severe cramps than for the chronic arthritis patient. Nonetheless, as with other drugs, side effects do occur in some women.

Prescription of these drugs is avoided in pregnant women and discontinued when women complain of allergic reactions, gastrointestinal side effects, and/or nervous disorders. Some women cannot take aspirin for the same reasons. It is also a prostaglandin inhibitor. Newer drugs are being tested, however, with lower risk and fewer side effects, and a higher therapeutic benefit to the patient.

"Prostaglandins, culprits in cramps,
are tied to endometriosis-infertility"

The theory that prostaglandins are related to infertility caused by endometriosis was recently reported in *Medical World News*. Dr. Terrance S. Drake, head of reproductive biology at the National Medical Center, studied infertile women with endometriosis and found great volumes of peritoneal fluid with high levels of prostaglandin-breakdown elements. He surmises that the prostaglandins block conception and suggests their suppression with aspirin. He described his theory to The American Fertility Society. He and his colleagues collected peritoneal fluid from sixty-six women undergoing laparoscopy. They found significantly more fluid in the thirty-two women with endometriosis, with the largest amounts in women with the most severe cases. Prostaglandins in the peritoneal cavity have also been discovered to inhibit conception in laboratory animals.

It is an interesting theory: an aspirin a day keeps endometriosis at bay (and might improve the chances for fertility). For now, however, the prostaglandin theory is just one of many.

Why does Dr. Drake recommend aspirin and not Motrin or a stronger prostaglandin inhibitor? He doubts the Food and Drug Administration "would let me give such drugs during the menstrual cycle because they aren't recommended during gestation." What he would like to do is to compare the effects of powerful prostaglandin inhibitors with those of danazol, the miracle drug (a steroid) currently advocated for the effective treatment of endometriosis.

THE THERAPEUTIC BABY

A woman who has just been told that she has endometriosis may ask, "What do I do?" "Well, you could have a baby. It will get rid of the endometriosis," her gynecologist may tell her. In fact, the latest edition of *Gynecology and Obstetrics*, edited by John Sciarra and used in medical schools across the country, advocates, "If the [endometriosis] patient is married, early pregnancy is suggested, and the patient is advised to have subsequent pregnancies as quickly as is economically sound."

In such a circumstance, the woman who does not want to get pregnant may want to search for another gynecologist. If she wants children, fine, let her try it. But having children will not *cure* endometriosis. Women in their twenties with endometriosis may have a child, but eventually the endometriosis can return (on an average of seven years later). In other words, those women who do not have an early pregnancy often show symptoms seven years earlier than women who do become pregnant. In addition, studies indicate that 20 percent of all endometriosis patients have had at least one child.

Dr. Ernest Nora, head of obstetrics at Columbus Hospital in Chicago, says, "Pregnancy is a possible preventative measure, but obviously it isn't for everyone and it's not a sure preventative."

During pregnancy there is an increase in estrogen and progesterone, which in turn suppresses pituitary secretion of gonadotrophin, causing amenorrhea and anovulation (cessation of menstruation and ovulation). Also, there is a transformation of the endometrial lining of the uterus. So endometriosis usually does regress while the woman is pregnant.

One endometriosis victim, Diane Karnes, tells her story in *Prevention*. "I started having second thoughts about having a child," she says. "I realized my decision was made in desperation, and I just could not have a baby to cure an illness."

Many gynecologists have come to the same conclusion, although rather late in the game. A shaky marriage can become even shakier when a couple is pressured into an unwanted pregnancy. To have a child every three or four years in order to prevent endometriosis is not economically feasible for most couples today.

The "therapeutic baby" still is being promoted, although it is fast losing credibility. The country has changed. Women have changed. Once upon a time large families helped out on the farm. They're no longer needed down on the condominium.

To be a mother has become a choice. Today a woman might marry someone who brings a family with him. Now, she can take the Pill until she is ready. In fact, many doctors have already turned to the Pill at least to forestall endometriosis in their younger patients. If the Pill is used to effect pseudopregnancy (see pp. 78–85), often the condition will recede in milder cases.

We have come a long way from the "therapeutic baby."

PART TWO

TREATMENTS

6

*Laparoscopy
and Other
Methods for Diagnosis*

DOCTORS VARY FROM conservative to ultraconservative. For the most part, they have been taught not to jump into a diagnosis. Today, miraculous diagnostic tools using sound waves, x-rays, and light-optic sources are available to reduce the chance of human error. Doctors rely on these new technological devices to confirm findings from the office examination. Some doctors may wait awhile. Others may take advantage of the newly purchased mammography machine or endoscope and recommend diagnostic procedures right away. They reason that the patient should have the benefit of technology sooner or later, so why not sooner?

Dr. Arnold Relman, editor of the prestigious *New England Journal of Medicine*, has lectured often about medical care as commerce in America. He laments this trend, citing the readiness of insurance companies to pay for expensive diagnostic tests, especially when the underutilized machines are available.

In a typical visit, a woman in whom mild endometriosis is suspected may be the victim of consumer medicine. The doctor may suggest that she have a mammography, an endometrial biopsy, a hysteroscopy, a laparoscopy, and a D&C, and she may be encouraged not to malinger a moment longer.

"LET'S WAIT AND SEE"

In contrast, doctors trained in the more traditional school of medicine will want to take their time to observe the patient and the progress of the disease before prescribing useless and often expensive tests. One sourcebook calls this management of endometriosis "studied neglect."

Observation will be the more likely course if the case is mild and the pelvic exam has revealed only slight tenderness and a few nodules not implicating the ovaries. "Expectant treatment" can be helpful, although some doctors do not consider observation a treatment. Dr. Robert Kistner of Harvard believes, "Reassurance and mild analgesics are adequate for such patients [with mild cases]."

If the physician suspects mild endometriosis, subsequent pelvic exams should be scheduled at least every six months to follow the progress (or regression) of the disease.

What does the patient do during this "let's wait and see" period? Mild endometriosis can produce severe pain. If so, she will probably leave the doctor's office with a prescription for painkillers. Beware of the doctor who sends a woman away with painkillers and nothing else—no definite scheduled appointment, no talk of further treatment, no reassurance that this, too, will pass. Painkillers are addictive and do not always work.

The patient has a right (an obligation, in fact) to know what will happen if the painkillers do not work, if her symptoms continue, if she cannot get past the receptionist when she needs reassurance.

The ideal doctor who suspects mild endometriosis will

- follow the patient closely
- ask her to record her symptoms in relationship to her menstrual cycle
- recommend a mild analgesic first with the suggestion that she call for a stronger analgesic if the pain is not alleviated

- make a future appointment while she is still in the office, preferably three months and no more than six months away
- encourage her to call if the symptoms worsen or are not relieved, and
- explain what the next step of her treatment will be.

Let us say that several months have elapsed and reassurance and aspirin have done very little for the woman. Dr. Paul Manganiello of the Dartmouth-Hitchcock Medical Center says, "A lot of times you don't just jump into laparoscopy. You can try to see if you can treat endometriosis medically. When a woman is cycled with birth-control pills where we do see an artificial period, oftentimes the pain doesn't go away from endometriosis. If I had a teenager on birth-control pills and she was still having pain, I would be very suspicious and would consider laparoscopy. Another medication is Motrin. But there are patients who have endometriosis who don't respond to Motrin."

Motrin is a prostaglandin inhibitor prescribed for primary dysmenorrhea (menstrual cramping with no apparent organic cause). According to the book *Freedom from Menstrual Cramps*, drugs such as Motrin "provide relief from menstrual cramps in about 80% of all women with dysmenorrhea." Often these inhibitors are not very helpful for pain from endometriosis.

How popular is expectant treatment? In a recent *Mademoiselle* article on endometriosis, Drs. Arthur and Stuart Frank write, "Most women with endometriosis can be successfully treated with a careful examination, a complete explanation, some comforting reassurance, and occasional mild or moderate pain medications like aspirin or codeine when symptoms are present."

The length of time doctors and patients agree to wait can also be affected by the age of the woman. If she is young and doesn't want a family right away, she may decide to try the doctor's approach, especially if the symptoms do not restrict her normal life-style.

The older woman may choose to wait for menopause, when the ovarian hormones diminish, causing the symptoms to subside and the condition to regress. From age thirty-five or so until fifty, however, is a long time to support a condition, especially with symptoms of pain and irregular bleeding. For peace of mind, the woman might choose to have a laparoscopy and biopsy, even though the doctor assures her that her case is mild. The waiting approach may seem easier for her when the diagnosis is substantiated by laparoscopy.

When is waiting not advisable? If severe endometriosis of the ovaries is found during the pelvic exam, the pain is incapacitating, bleeding is profuse, or all symptoms progressively worsen, it is time to act!

SOME DIAGNOSTIC PROCEDURES TO DETECT
ENDOMETRIOSIS IN VARIOUS PARTS OF THE BODY

Procedure	Location of Endometriosis
Renogram (x-ray of the kidney shadow following the injection of radiopaque medium)	ureter
Pyelogram (radiographic visualization of the kidneys and the area around them)	kidneys
Cystoscopy and cystoscopic biopsy (light scope permits visualization, biopsy, and photography)	bladder, ureter, kidneys
Chest x-rays and/or	chest

Procedure	Location of Endometriosis
Thoracentesis (a needle is inserted in the lungs and liquid withdrawn to examine for possible endometrial blood in the chest)	
Pelvic exam (to find cysts, nodules, displaced reproductive organs, and/or tumor of the bladder, which appears in a great many cases)	pelvic area
Biopsy (microscopic examination of tissue, performed in the laboratory) and/or Culdoscopy (a light scope is passed through the vagina)	lesions of perineum, vagina, cervix
Sigmoidoscopy and biopsy (uses the light scope inserted in the rectum to visualize the bowel and look for bleeding, obstruction, and abnormalities; a biopsy is performed to determine if malignancy is present) and/or Barium enema (shows deformities in the intestine; two should be performed, one early in the cycle, another at menstruation)	bowel
Laparoscopy (most areas may be visualized by the laparoscope inserted at the navel)	uterus, tubes, ovaries, and several other organs, including rectal sacral area, appendix

Womancare recommends that if a woman "decides to accept treatment on the basis of presumptive diagnosis, she should be convinced that the risks and expense of laparoscopy outweigh the risks and expense of undergoing possibly unnecessary hormone therapy." Most doctors will not prescribe prolonged hormone treatment without verification of the condition by biopsy and laparoscopy.

LAPAROSCOPY AND BIOPSY

The precursor of the modern laparoscope can probably be attributed to Dr. Kalk, a German who devised a system of lenses with a viewing angle of 135 degrees. In 1929, Dr. H. Kalk performed a hundred pelvic examinations on women with his new invention. In 1952, Gladu Fourestier and his colleagues developed a method of transmitting light along a quartz rod from the near to the far end of a telescope. Prior to this time, lamps were used to look into the pelvic area. With the new quartz endoscope, photographs could be taken without the danger of electrical failure or overheating.

The standard laparoscope used in hospitals today is a refinement of these earlier endoscopes. The laparoscope gained popularity in the United States from 1968 on, with the additional benefit of fiber optics. In the current laparoscope, light travels a network of thin glass threads through a flexible tube.

The endoscope today is a multipurpose tool. It not only allows the doctor to visualize the inner recesses of the body, but also permits photographing and biopsy. Laparoscopy has become the diagnostic procedure most doctors rely on to confirm suspicions of endometriosis. It enables them to visually check virtually all areas where the endometrial implants might have spread.

Different optic scopes are used depending on where the endometriosis is suspected.

Risk

Dr. J. A. Chalmers, author of one of the extremely few medical texts written in English entirely on the subject of endometriosis (now out of print), observes that culdoscopy—passing the light scope through the vagina—carries the risk of a perforated bowel and that if the cul-de-sac is full of endometriosis, visualization often proves impossible. More and more doctors agree and choose laparoscopy and/or hysteroscopy (endoscopic examination of the interior of the uterus) for the visualization of endometriosis.

A survey of risk factors for diagnostic laparoscopy places the complication rate at about five out of one thousand procedures. This figure includes less serious complications such as skin infections. Serious perforations involve about two out of one thousand laparoscopic procedures.

Cost

Office diagnostic procedures are much less costly than those done on a patient in a hospital. For example, colposcopy is a fairly recent office procedure whereby the gynecologist looks through a binocular-type instrument to detect abnormalities of the cervix, take a biopsy, and see into the vagina. It is helpful in diagnosing endometriosis of the cervix.

Both hysteroscopy and laparoscopy may be performed on an outpatient basis. Some hospitals, however, only permit laparoscopy on an overnight basis. When the gynecologist suggests laparoscopy, the patient should inquire whether or not it will be performed on an in- or outpatient basis. Contrary to what some doctors may suggest to the patient, laparoscopy may be performed on an outpatient basis.

Dr. Jaroslav Marik, director of the University of California School of Medicine in Los Angeles, says, "When the procedure is done in-hospital, the costs run much higher . . ." These rates vary from hospital to hospital, but the cost of outpatient versus inpatient laparoscopy can be double and sometimes triple.

If the gynecologist performs laparoscopy only on an inpatient basis, the patient may ask for a recommendation of someone who will perform it on an outpatient basis, especially if she has minimum insurance coverage.

Laparoscopy

A laparoscopy is referred to as Band-Aid surgery or belly-button surgery because the laparoscope is inserted at the navel, leaving an imperceptible scar.

The patient admitted to the hospital will be administered general anesthesia. A tube attached to a machine that breathes for her is placed in her throat. Then the woman is given a pelvic exam. If a D&C has been ordered, this will be performed first. The cervix is dilated and the uterus aspirated or scraped with a curette. Next, a needle is pushed through the skin right at the fold of the belly button, and carbon dioxide is pumped into the belly. This gas causes the organs to separate so they may be visualized.

The surgeon pushes a trocar (an instrument about eight inches long with a pyramid-shaped end) through a half-inch incision just below the navel. The trocar is surrounded with a fiberglass sleeve. A hose fits into the valve of the sleeve and a machine pumps more CO_2 into the abdomen to replace any that leaks out. The trocar is then removed from the sleeve and the laparoscope (eighteen inches long and about half an inch in diameter) is substituted.

The patient is tilted backward so that her head points toward the floor. This causes the intestines to fall against the chest cavity so that the Fallopian tubes and ovaries may be observed.

Sometimes a second incision is made above the pubic hair to view the lower abdomen. The light from the scope shines through the belly much like a flashlight held to the hand.

There may be three sets of instruments in the patient at one time. First, of course, is the laparoscope. The instruments in the vagina include a tenaculum or surgical hook attached to the cervix, which in turn is attached to a long, thin instrument called a cannula. The cannula goes into the opening of the cervix. These may be used to manipulate the uterus during the operation.

Conservative surgery may be performed during the laparoscopy if the endometriosis implants are not extensive or severe. The surgeon may also run dye through the Fallopian tubes to see if they are blocked.

After the operation, the gas is forced out of the abdomen much like deflating a rubber ball. The incisions usually bleed very little. They are either stapled or sewn with stitches that dissolve. The patient may have to vomit. She is placed on her side so that she will not be able to draw up any of the contents from her intestines into her lungs.

Afterward, she is taken to the recovery room, and when the doctor is sure there are no complications, she returns to her hospital room.

The same stages for recovery apply to laparoscopy as to most surgery. The tube that was placed in the throat may cause soreness, and the anesthesia itself can cause nausea. It will be difficult to walk because of abdominal soreness, and the patient will probably be on an IV (intravenous) solution for several hours. She will have difficulty urinating and may have discomfort in her shoulders as a result of the carbon dioxide gas gravitating there when she was tilted on the operating table. The patient also may have some bleeding from the vagina, especially if a D&C was performed.

Although laparoscopy is lightly referred to as Band-Aid surgery, it is nevertheless surgery. Women might want to consider taking high doses (5000–6000 mg) of vitamin C prior to admittance to the hospital. Some doctors do not concur that vitamin C combats infection, others recommend large doses. Women should make sure they are not tired or run down. Usually, there will be no complications, and the hospital stay rarely exceeds two days.

Outpatient Laparoscopy

Outpatient laparoscopy does not mean half an hour in the doctor's office, but the patient will often be able to go home from the surgical facility the same day that the operation is performed.

The procedure itself is the same as for an inpatient. The patient is taken to the holding area near the operating room and an intravenous infusion is started. Shaving of body hair, as for other operations, is usually unnecessary.

The American College of Obstetricians and Gynecologists states in an information booklet: "If the procedure is to be done under a local anesthesia, the patient is given medication to help her relax when she arrives in the operating room, and the anesthetic injection is given." Under general anesthesia, by contrast, the patient is given an injection to put her to sleep, and then the gas is administered.

The booklet also states, "Most women are ready to leave the hospital two to four hours after the procedure." It does not mention having a friend or spouse available to drive the patient home and help her to bed. Most women will feel like they have been through an ordeal and will need a strong arm to lean on.

Dr. Anne Ward of the Michael Reese Hospital in Chicago says, however, that most physicians demand general anesthesia for outpatient laparoscopy. She states that the procedure could become "exceedingly dangerous under a local anesthesia if the patient starts to move while the trocar is being inserted."

One concerned husband who stayed with his wife in the outpatient recovery room of a large hospital in Boston told the author that at least ten women were there for outpatient laparoscopy, and not one of them felt up to leaving a few hours after surgery. In fact, he wished he had kept his wife there overnight, since they had a two-hour drive back to New Hampshire. Even though he was there to help, she felt groggy and sick.

He commented that several of the women were there because of endometriosis. Many of these women thought that laparoscopy was surgical treatment and that they would be cured when they went home. It should be understood that laparoscopy is a *diagnostic* procedure, unless the doctor indicates otherwise. Sometimes, a few accessible implants may be removed, but the procedure is usually exploratory, to see if endometriosis exists and how extensive it is.

Before and After Laparoscopy

Laparoscopy and D&C are common, low-risk diagnostic surgical procedures. If a woman knows what to expect, some of the more stressful aspects can be alleviated and her fears assuaged.

The patient will be asked to come to the hospital with an empty stomach. She will be given an enema to make sure that her intestines are clean. A chest x-ray, ECG (electrocardiogram, which records heart function), blood tests, and medical history including allergies will probably be scheduled. She will also be asked to bathe to cut down as much as possible the skin's normal bacterial count before the operation.

The woman undergoing anesthesia should be permitted to talk with the anesthesiologist and ask what anesthetic will be used. If she has any fears or objections, these should be resolved beforehand. She may also ask to talk with her own gynecologist-surgeon if she needs information or reassurance. The surgeon may not always be available, but should see the patient sometime before surgery.

Afterward, as mentioned, there will be soreness, light vaginal bleeding, nausea, mild tenderness around the incisions, and possibly some bleeding from the incisions. These discomforts may disappear fairly soon; in some women they take up to a week to disappear.

Avoid tight clothes. Tight-waisted jeans are not the thing to wear on a trip to the hospital for laparoscopy. A waistless dress or smock will feel much better over the tender incisions. The incisions may be black and blue at first, later turning yellow (which means they are healing). After bathing or showering, pat them dry. Avoid lifting anything that weighs more than a few pounds for at least a week.

The patient should check with her doctor regarding when sexual relations may be resumed. Tampons, feminine hygiene sprays, and vaginal suppositories should not be used for two weeks.

Menstruation will probably begin about four weeks after a D&C, and should start at its normal time after a laparoscopy. Fever, swelling, cramps, foul-smelling discharge, heavy bleeding, or missing the next period after a six- to eight-week wait indicate that the doctor should be notified immediately.

Biopsy

A biopsy is the excision of tissue for examination under the microscope. While the laparoscopy is being performed, the surgeon will take samples of tissue from the endometrial lining of the uterus (endometrial biopsy) and also from any implants, cysts, tumors, or other suspicious-looking growths in the pelvic area. Specimens are sent directly to the pathology laboratory for examination and report.

CHOCOLATE CYSTS AND POWDER BURNS

Surgeons wax poetic when describing what endometriosis looks like in the human body.

Color

One doctor describes recently formed lesions as "pink in color." Thus they have been dubbed "raspberry and mulberry spots." The pinkish spots are commonly found in the uterosacral area. Blue "powder-burn" spots of endometriosis may be found on the ovaries and elsewhere. Surgeons sometimes refer to them as "chocolate cysts." Some doctors think that they look like "blood blisters." In the course of time, the blood in these cysts becomes thick, tarry, and dark brown. Dr. Kistner of Harvard cautions that "not all chocolate cysts are endometriosis," and a biopsy should be performed to determine the nature of the cyst.

In the vagina and on the cervix, blue powder-burns have been described as "firm bluish domelike bulges" and on pelvic tissue as "blueberry spots."

Texture

Endometriomas (large cysts) are firm and hard. During their active stage they look thick and velvety. As the scar tissue builds, they may adhere to other organs, becoming fibrous in appearance. During pregnancy or hormone treatment, the lesions may look gelatinous. Just before or during menopause, some of the implants pucker into white scars. One doctor advises looking for "puckered nodules."

Size

On the ovaries (which are involved in approximately 60 percent of all endometriosis cases), the implants may be as small as a pinhead or grow and coalesce into a cyst the size of a grapefruit. Active endometriomas swell and increase in size during menstruation, and then usually recede. "Webby" endometriosis is an elusive, spreading scar-tissue system that entangles and snags the uterus and often the broad and round ligaments that support it.

Stroma

The Greek word literally means bed or foundation. In chocolate cysts, mulberry spots, or whatever one wants to call them, the part that bleeds is the stroma.

If punctured, the endometrioma will produce "altered blood," or tarry, dark-brown blood. The spillage from a large punctured endometrioma into the peritoneal cavity can cause great havoc.

In summary, to the trained surgeon's eye, some types of implants, lesions, and cysts may be easily identified as typical endometriosis. But it must be emphasized that not all endometriosis can be distinguished from other tumors, cysts, and abnormal growths. The only sure diagnosis is by *combined visualization* and *biopsy*.

Nor can it be overstated that laparoscopy must be performed by an experienced laparoscopist. Rupture of large ovarian endometriomas may be fatal. Even the accidental prodding of smaller implants may spread the tissue into other parts of a woman's body. Biopsy should be as carefully executed as possible.

ULTRASOUND

Sonar was being developed and refined during World War II for the detection of enemy submarines. Scientists experimented by bouncing high-frequency vibrations off body masses to construct a position and locate an object unseen by the naked eye. Similarly, ultrasound used in hospitals is a highly developed method of visualizing the interior of the body. It is commonly used in pregnancy to monitor the fetus, determine the exact position of the baby in the uterus, and observe contractions in labor. It may also be used to locate a "lost" IUD or to visualize any abnormalities on the ovaries.

Ultrasound is painless. The sound waves are targeted at the body via a microphonelike device. The waves bounce back in echo patterns that appear in the form of a picture on a screen.

Some women worry that ultrasound might involve risk, although most doctors claim that the risk is much greater with diagnostic x-rays, and that ultrasound is perfectly harmless. Nevertheless, ultrasound is one of those new diagnostic tools that every hospital must have, and testing as to its safety has been minimal.

"How could it possibly hurt you?" some women ask. "It's only sound waves. Every time you turn on the radio you're dealing with sound waves. We're surrounded by radio waves." One might reply that those sound waves are being directed at random from a transmitter, not at close range and in high frequencies at a woman's body.

Although little research has been done on the advantages or disadvantages of ultrasound, a study in 1973 revealed some interesting facts. Changes in the amniotic fluid (nutrient fluid surrounding the fetus in the uterus) were found in sixty-five fluid specimens taken from women exposed to ultrasonic monitoring, and 60 percent of those specimens failed to grow in the laboratory. Only 12 percent of the specimens failed to grow in the control group of pregnant women *not* exposed to ultrasound.

In his book *Mal(e)practice: How Doctors Manipulate Women*, Dr. Robert Mendelsohn questions the use of fetal monitors and states, "Investigators also have found delayed neurological development, altered emotional and behavioral effects, fetal abnormalities, and blood and vascular changes in animals exposed to ultrasound."

More frequently, doctors are turning to ultrasound to diagnose cysts and tumors. One patient from Connecticut who had three cysts and internal bleeding was examined by ultrasound, which showed a cyst on her bladder. It turned out to be endometriosis. Ultrasound was used on another interviewee from Massachusetts in order to monitor the ovaries in case other cysts appeared.

One recent study used ultrasound preoperatively on sixty patients with tumors of the ovary in order to differentiate whether they were malignant or benign. In 90 percent of the cases, diagnosis by ultrasound proved correct. The researcher recommended that ultrasound be used more often for this sort of diagnosis.

Another study was conducted in which the researcher tried to diagnose endometriosis with ultrasonic equipment and found it impossible to distinguish endometriosis from cystic lesions and PID without doing a laparoscopy and a biopsy as well.

Perhaps the results from a study at the State University of New York Downstate Medical Center sums up the advantages and disadvantages of the use of ultrasound for diagnosing endometriosis: "Ultrasonography helps in the identification and localization of pelvic masses, but is not specific." In other words, if the captain knows there's an enemy submarine in the region, and it's not the time for whale migration, he might have something.

Thus far, ultrasound seems most beneficial postsurgically or after hormone treatment in order to record the progression or regression of the condition. Today, ultrasound has been accepted and its advantages touted in the diagnostic field.

X-rays, however, especially of the reproductive organs, carry known risk; unless they are prescribed for a definite treatment such as the remission of cancer cells, or the castration of a woman where surgery is not possible, they are not recommended on a regular diagnostic basis.

7

Medical Treatment:
Hormones

MOST DOCTORS ARE less certain about the causes of endometriosis than about what seems to make it go away. In a woman's body they have observed two processes that cause endometriosis to recede and sometimes stop altogether. One is pregnancy. But doctors and women alike have come to the conclusion that pregnancy every few years does not provide a practical solution, or, for that matter, a definite cure.

The other process is menopause. As a woman's hormonal system winds down and less estrogen is produced in the ovaries, endometriosis automatically regresses. The woman stops menstruating and the endometrial implants stop bleeding too.

Nobody need tell the reader that the United States has become the leading nation for the manufacture of synthetic hormones. We have distributed the Pill on a worldwide basis; each company has a different formula to offer. The upshot is that today we have hormones that cause what doctors call pseudopregnancy (see p. 78). They are referred to as "female" hormones and include estrogen, progesten, or a combination of both, which naturally occur in a woman's body. We also have pills that can cause pseudomenopause (see pp. 85-91). These are "male" hormones derived from testosterone, which is produced in the male reproductive system and only in small amounts in women.

Doctors have gravitated to treatment by hormones for a number of menstrual disorders in addition to prescribing them as contraceptives.

What hormones are prescribed for endometriosis? Each doctor has his or her own regimen of treatment, but most agree that surgery, especially radical surgery, must be resorted to for severe endometriosis. Some doctors think, as we have noted, that mild endometriosis will disappear of its own accord. Others might prescribe a cycle of hormones, then wait to see if symptoms disappear.

Moderate endometriosis might involve a different approach —that is, conservative surgery followed by six to nine months of hormones. Hormones will often be the treatment of choice, especially if the woman desires pregnancy.

Doctors tend to recommend hysterectomy for severe cases of endometriosis, especially in a woman who does not plan on children and is thirty-five or older.

These are general guidelines and are apt to vary from doctor to doctor. Most of the medical literature, however, points to observation in milder cases, combined hormones or conservative surgery (sometimes both) in mild to moderate cases, and radical surgery in severe cases implicating the ovaries.

PSEUDOPREGNANCY (Combination Hormones)

"My doctor told me to get pregnant, and I didn't even have a boyfriend," one endometriosis patient lamented. Doctors confronted by endometriosis patients who do not wish to become pregnant may consider placing them on the Pill. The Pill simulates pregnancy without the baby because the hormones suppress ovulation and menstruation. Many side effects that women experience from the Pill and resultant pseudo-pregnancy are the same as those in pregnancy.

What are these hormones? One gynecologist, Dr. Herbert Niles, in a paper titled "The Hormonal Aspects of Endometriosis," writes: "Prior to 1957, estrogens in the form of diethyl-Stilbestrol (DES) were the treatment for endometriosis in large doses." After several thousands of cases of uterine cancer appeared in the daughters of mothers who had been given DES for a number of problems during pregnancy, DES lost considerable popularity.

As a result, combined progesten-estrogen therapy has become the most common pseudopregnancy regimen today. More than twenty-five different preparations of combined hormones are on the market.

COMBINATION HORMONES SPECIFICALLY
INDICATED FOR ENDOMETRIOSIS

Brand	FDA Approved	Dosage
Enovid (Searle)	Yes	5 mg. only, daily for two weeks with increments up to 20 mg. daily for 6–9 months beginning day 5 of menstrual cycle.
Norlutin (Parke-Davis)	Yes	10 mg. for 2 weeks with increments until 30 mg. per day is reached, continue from 6–9 months.
Norlutate (Parke-Davis)	Yes	5 mg. with increments of 2.5 mg. per day every 2 weeks until 15 mg. per day is reached.

OTHER COMBINATION HORMONES (NOT FDA
APPROVED) FOR ENDOMETRIOSIS

Bevicon	Norlestrin
Demulen	Norlestrin FE
Enovid-E	Ortho-Novum
Loestrin	Ovcon
Lo/Ovral	Ovral
Modicon	Ovulen
Norinyl	Zorane

Possible Side Effects*

Possible side effects of hormones include nausea, cramps, edema (bloating), breakthrough bleeding, infertility after the Pill cycle, breast tenderness, weight gain, headaches, acne, vaginal itching, vaginal infection, despondency and depression, nervousness, dizziness, eye cataracts, altered sex drive, change in appetite, and hair loss.

Contraindications

Women who smoke, who are pregnant, or who have liver conditions, a history of cardiovascular disease, blood clots, or undiagnosed bleeding should be cautious about taking hormones.

Drug Interactions

Pill effectiveness may be decreased by barbiturates, ampicillin, phenylbutazone, phenytoin (Dilantin), and rifampin.

* Compiled from Harold Silverman and Simon Gilbert, *The Pill Book* (Bantam, 1979), 230 pp. These apply to oral contraceptives listed above.

FDA Approval

Why are only three or four of the many oral contraceptives approved by the FDA for endometriosis? One FDA official suggested that approval often tends to be an involved, costly process for the drug companies.

For example, Searle has tested Enovid for endometriosis, but their other products, Enovid-E, Ovulen, and Demulen have not been approved for treating this condition. Testing takes years of research, first by the company and then by the FDA.

Liken hormones to cereals. Kellogg manufactures sugar-coated corn flakes, plain corn flakes, flakes with raisins. They're all more or less the same, but targeted toward different customers. Similar reasons apply to brands of combination hormones. If a doctor thinks a certain oral contraceptive will work for the endometriosis patient, it will be prescribed, regardless of FDA approval.

Side Effects

Some combined hormones contain more estrogen than others. The consumer-patient must be aware that she will be taking much more than the ordinary "contraceptive" dose of the Pill. In fact, she might be taking up to eight Pills a day!

One depressed woman interviewed in Boston said that she was up to forty milligrams a day. "I've gained twenty-five pounds," she confided. Her surgeon (who had already removed an ovarian cyst) was attempting to preserve her fertility and keep the endometriosis in check.

Another woman said, "The treatment they put me on in 1972 was massive doses of hormones. I was taking fifteen times the ordinary dosage for the daily birth-control pill. It produced severe depression."

Anyone who decides to follow hormone therapy should read Barbara and Gideon Seaman's informative book *Women and the Crisis in Sex Hormones*, especially the chapters on side effects and on recovering from the Pill. The woman with endometriosis will probably take the Pill on a noncyclic basis —without interruption for six to nine months. The dose will be much greater than for contraceptive purposes, and thus the side effects will most likely be greater.

Often the doctor will prescribe iron supplements to ward off anemia. The Seamans, however, advocate taking carefully selected vitamins as well, since the Pill depletes normal supplies. They refer to one patient, Robin, treated for endometriosis with Enovid. Her husband says, "When Robin is taking Enovid, I have to walk with her slowly, like an old man. When she's off it, I have to run to keep up." But Robin's endometriosis acts up if she does not take Enovid. So for her, and many women like her, it is either the devil or the deep blue sea.

Risks

In a discussion about hormone therapy recorded in the journal *Patient Care*, the doctors were asked when combined hormones would be contraindicated. Dr. Russell Malinak of Baylor Medical College in Houston answered, "[In] the presence of a well-defined ovarian endometrioma." He went on to explain that hormones tend to enlarge, soften, and consequently lead to the rupture of such endometriomas.

For this reason, there is a running controversy among surgeons about using hormones prior to surgery for endometriosis. Some surgeons feel that the hormones enlarge the endometriosis implants, soften them, and thus facilitate surgery. Others are emphatically opposed to this approach because of the risk of rupture and subsequent spreading of the condition.

Risks from taking hormones must be carefully weighed against the risks of other treatments. Naturally, some women question the safety of the birth-control pill, especially since four to eight pills per day are often recommended. When asked what the doctors would say if their patients voiced concern, one doctor responded that he tells these women that the death rate associated with Pill use is three per hundred thousand, as opposed to twenty-seven per hundred thousand for automobile use.

The analogy is a bit far-fetched, since the Pill is not exactly a hit-and-run accident. DES cancer victims started turning up twenty years after administration of the hormone to their mothers. Doctors often quote statistics of fatality as the only viable proof for showing concern.

At first, the choice of the Pill versus conservative surgery may seem obvious. The Pill is less expensive, and a woman need not take time to recover. She just pops it into her mouth and swallows. But if nausea comes on and the patient must miss work, or if she gains weight or becomes extremely depressed, she might decide on alternative treatment.

Which Combination?

Each pill has a different ratio of estrogen. The estrogen is added in order to prevent breakthrough bleeding. Enovid currently seems to be the pill of choice. It is highly progestational with minimal estrogen. Nausea may be overcome through increasing the dosage gradually and building up tolerance.

If the woman has fibroids and endometriosis, her fibroids will grow with estrogen. Thus, when fibroids have been diagnosed along with endometriosis, Depo-Provera will sometimes be prescribed. Depo-Provera is a progestational hormone given by injection. It is not advised for women wishing to become pregnant, however, because ovulation often is suppressed well after the treatment has been discontinued. Progestens such as Depo-Provera are extremely potent and are prescribed only when other hormones would be contraindicated.

Another warning must be acknowledged when the doctor prescribes Depo-Provera. The general cancer rate of the female population is thirty-six per hundred thousand women. With Depo-Provera the rate is 235 per hundred thousand women, according to Upjohn Laboratories research. But the FDA's testing revealed 410 per hundred thousand women. Obviously, the cancer risks of this hormone are much higher than for combination hormones.

Recurrence and Conception Rates

Hormones rarely cure moderate to severe endometriosis and thus are often not prescribed in these cases, unless as a diagnostic tool or where surgery involves greater risk.

Hormones have proven useful and effective in mild cases of endometriosis. They may alleviate symptoms and cause the condition to recede in the early stages. And in particular, they may be the treatment of choice in teenagers with mild endometriosis. Where pain is the main symptom and fertility is not in question, the doctor may prescribe hormones without laparoscopy on a cyclic basis (every twenty-one days) rather than the usual heavy, noninterrupted dosage.

Conception subsequent to hormone treatment varies, but in stages I and II endometriosis (surface endometriosis without endometriomas of tubo-ovarian adhesions), Dr. Robert Kistner at Harvard established a 50 percent pregnancy rate after combined hormonal therapy on 186 patients. Other researchers have found the average to be between 25 percent and 75 percent.

Dr. W. P. Dmowski, author of a chapter on endometriosis from the *Obstetrics & Gynecology Annual*, 1981, summarizes the likelihood of a complete and total cure either by hormone treatment or conservative surgery. "It should be emphasized," he writes, "that regardless of the method of treatment, the mechanism through which endometriosis developed in the particular patient has not been changed, and for that reason the recurrence of the disease is likely."

ENDOMETRIOSIS: PREGNANCY RATES—HORMONAL

Author of Study	Year	Therapy	No. of Patients	Pregnancy (%)
Jones	1962	Testosterone	28	10.0
Riva	1962	Estrogen + progesten	132	72.0
Gunning	1967	Depo-Provera	14	28.5
Williams	1967	Estrogen + progesten	44	72.0
Chambers	1968	Estrogen + progesten	55	26.5
Snaith	1968	Estrogen + progesten	28	25.0
Andrews	1974	Estrogen + progesten	7	43.0
Greenblatt	1974	Danazol	21	42.8
Kistner	1975	Estrogen + progesten	186	50.8

From *Clinical Gynecology*, a reprint, vol. 1, chap. 38, p. 26. From R. W. Kistner, M.D. "Endometriosis," in *Gynecology and Obstetrics*, vol. 1, ed. by John Sciarra (Philadelphia: Harper & Row, 1980).

PSEUDOMENOPAUSE (Danazol)

Androgens are "male" hormones secreted in the male testes, which control secondary sex characteristics such as body hair and deepening of the voice. When administered to women, the same changes may occur. Male sex hormones are thought to block pituitary stimulation of the ovaries and the production of LH (lutinizing hormones) and FSH (follicle-stimulating hormones). Danazol is a synthetic androgen.

Some call danazol a "miracle" drug. It was approved by the FDA for the treatment of endometriosis in 1976. To date, it has been tested for about twelve years. In the United States danazol is manufactured by Winthrop Laboratories under the brand name Danocrine. In Canada it is called Cyclomen.

How Danazol Works

Although the term "pseudomenopause" is currently in use, a *British Medical Journal* editorial suggests that this is inappropriate since ovulation does occur, although peaks in the hormone cycle do not. The editorial also states that gonadotropin concentrations remain normal. The *Medical Letter* (an industry newsletter) reports, "Danazol *probably* acts by inhibiting the release of gonadotropins."

Winthrop Laboratories says Danocrine "suppresses ovarian estrogen and progesterone secretion and induces anovulation."

Research is still continuing, and one hopes that all medical sources will soon come to an understanding about how danazol works.

Benefits over Pseudopregnancy

In pseudopregnancy the symptoms of endometriosis usually worsen, causing softening of and increase in the endometrial tissue within the first three months (what would be a trimester in a normal pregnancy). With danazol treatment this does not occur. Danazol does not stimulate the natural body hormones but blocks and actually lowers natural hormone levels in the body. Instead of initial softening, there is a sort of atrophy of the endometriosis implants from the very first.

Side Effects

Unfortunately, as with the combined hormones, danazol also has its concomitant side effects. The largest number of complaints are of weight gain, muscle cramping, and decreased breast size. Sometimes there will be menopausal symptoms such as flushing and hot flashes, acne, growth and darkening of facial hair, and voice changes. Liver dysfunction, bloating (edema), enlargement of the clitoris, vaginitis, and vulvitis have also been reported. Some of these side effects may be irreversible.

Weight Gain

Dr. Paul Manganiello of the Dartmouth-Hitchcock Medical Center brings up an interesting point, especially for women concerned with weight gain. Androgens are anabolic. This means that they cause the synthesis of body proteins. Serious athletes often take anabolic compounds to build muscle tissue. The weight gain in progesten-estrogen combined hormone treatment is mostly due to water retention. This weight can be lost when treatment has been discontinued.

"Danocrine is anabolic," Dr. Manganiello says. "It's a different type of weight gain. It is actual protein retention, and probably a lot harder to get rid of."

It is interesting to note that edema or fluid retention occurs with danazol treatment too. But on the following chart, weight gain and muscle cramps are the two most common complaints. Anabolics effect a change in body muscle. This should be given consideration when considering the alternatives.

Cost

The high cost of Danocrine has been a definite disadvantage. Edward Cleary, pharmacist at the Village Pharmacy in Peterborough, New Hampshire, quotes a price of $131 for a bottle of one hundred capsules, and he underlines that Winthrop Laboratories will not give a refund on opened bottles. Thus, the customer must buy an entire bottle, even if she only needs a few more capsules to complete her treatment.

The current recommended dosage is 800 milligrams daily, although many doctors are finding that a lower dose is preferable. The capsules are 200 mg each. Four capsules daily for

SIDE EFFECTS REPORTED BY 71 ENDOMETRIOSIS PATIENTS
WHO COMPLETED 6 MONTHS OF DANAZOL THERAPY

	Mild	Moderate	Severe	Total
Weight gain				60 (85%)*
Muscle cramps	16 (23%)	17 (24%)	4 (6%)	37 (52%)
Decreased breast size	23 (32%)	9 (13%)	2 (3%)	34 (48%)
Flushing	13 (18%)	15 (21%)	2 (3%)	30 (42%)
Mood change	15 (21%)	10 (14%)	2 (3%)	27 (38%)
Oiliness, skin/hair	11 (15%)	12 (17%)	3 (4%)	26 (37%)
Depression	17 (24%)	5 (7%)	1 (1%)	23 (32%)
Sweating	12 (17%)	7 (10%)	4 (6%)	23 (32%)
Edema	7 (10%)	7 (10%)	4 (6%)	20 (28%)
Change in appetite	9 (13%)	11 (15%)	1 (1%)	20 (28%)
Acne	16 (23%)	3 (2%)	—	19 (27%)
Fatigue	11 (15%)	4 (6%)	—	18 (25%)
Growth of body hair	13 (18%)	2 (3%)	—	15 (21%)
Decreased sex drive	10 (14%)	3 (4%)	3 (4%)	14 (20%)
Nausea	8 (11%)	4 (6%)	—	12 (17%)
Headache	9 (13%)	3 (4%)	—	12 (17%)
Dizziness	6 (8%)	1 (1%)	—	7 (10%)
Insomnia	4 (6%)	2 (3%)	—	7 (10%)
Skin rash	3 (4%)	3 (4%)	—	6 (8%)
Increased sex drive	2 (3%)	3 (4%)	1 (1%)	6 (8%)
Deepening of voice	3 (4%)	2 (3%)	—	5 (7%)

* 0–1 lbs, 15%; 1–5 lbs, 22%; 6–10 lbs, 32%; 11–15 lbs, 18%; 16–20 lbs, 11%. (From V. C. Buttram, Jr., J. B. Belue, and R. Reiter, "Interim Report of a Study of Danazol for the Treatment of Endometriosis," *Fertility and Sterility* 37(1982): 478. Reproduced by permission of the publisher, The American Fertility Society, Birmingham, Ala.)

half a year (728 capsules) equals about 7¼ bottles at a cost of close to $1,000. Some sources quote prices of from $800 to $1,600 for six months of Danocrine. A few insurance companies will cover the cost of danazol treatment, others will not. If the doctor writes a letter for a Medicaid patient indicating treatment for endometriosis, the patient may be reimbursed. An official representing Medicaid says that danazol treatment is covered according to individual state regulations.

Contraindications

Danocrine should not be used if there is undiagnosed abnormal genital bleeding or impaired liver, kidney, or heart function; or if the woman is pregnant or breast feeding.

Recurrence and Conception Rates

In an interview, Dr. Robert Kistner of Harvard spoke about danazol: "It is an ideal temporary treatment, but danazol doesn't cure endometriosis. Danazol has certain side effects which in the lower doses aren't bad. One problem is that the recurrence rate is high, and another problem is that it doesn't get rid of ovarian endometriosis."

Clinical trials show that danazol usually is just as effective as or more effective than combined hormones in mild cases of endometriosis, but in severe cases danazol only proves partially effective.

Danazol is recommended in doses of 400 mg daily three months prior to surgery by many surgeons. They applaud its tendency to cause implants to atrophy, which makes surgery easier. Rupture becomes much less of a risk.

Several researchers have established the pregnancy rate subsequent to six to nine months of danazol treatment at 40 to 50 percent. Testing is ongoing, and results keep coming in. For women who would like to become pregnant but have a problem with infertility and endometriosis, danazol often can be successful. If pregnancy occurs, it will usually be from one to five months after therapy.

Recurrence rates of symptoms are high, however, and in one study with a six-year follow-up undertaken by one researcher, a 30 to 35 percent recurrence of endometriosis symptoms showed up three to four years after a three- to four-month course of danazol.

During danazol treatment of twenty patients in Finland, painful menstruation was relieved but returned somewhat reduced within ten months of the termination of treatment. Pelvic pain and painful defecation, however, disappeared and recurred only minimally after ten months. Other studies substantiate relief from symptoms for mild endometriosis, especially during treatment.

Pregnancy During Treatment

There have been reports of pregnancy while women were on danazol treatment. The treatment was discontinued, since danazol can have an androgenic (masculine) effect on the fetus.

It is advised that women on danazol resort to a nonhormonal contraceptive agent. Safe use of danazol during pregnancy has not been established.

Choosing Danazol Treatment

Not all results are in, but thus far researchers are optimistic. As with the birth-control pill, studies are zeroing in on the lowest effective dose that causes the least side effects. No woman wants to wake up a tenor with a five o'clock shadow on her chin. Many doctors are lowering the dose to minimize side effects.

Danazol is not a miracle cure for endometriosis, as some popular literature would have us believe. Some women see very little improvement. Diane Karnes, who told her story in

Prevention, found, "After four months of taking danazol . . . I noticed only a slight improvement in my condition." By contrast, one woman interviewed for this book who had severe endometriosis was ecstatic. Her doctor could find no remaining traces of the endometriosis subsequent to combined conservative surgery and danazol treatment.

Surgeons are prescribing six months of danazol preoperatively because excision of ovarian endometriosis is then easier and danazol tends to reduce adhesions at the site of surgery. Peritoneal endometriosis also responds to danazol treatment and danazol facilitates the surgeon's job since endometriosis surgery is sometimes difficult and involves a possible risk of rupture. Danazol therapy is commonly used postoperatively to clear up residual endometriosis and pave the way for pregnancy. Some doctors prefer danazol treatment prior to surgery only, thus allowing for pregnancy as soon as possible afterwards. Conservative surgery in combination with three to six months of danazol treatment offers a brighter future for women with a history of infertility and endometriosis. For many women the possible side effects and high cost of the drug have been well worth the returns: fertility and the chance to lead a healthy, normal life.

In short, hormone therapy with either a combined progesten-estrogen or with danazol must be discussed and assessed by the individual patient and her doctor.

8

Surgery:
Conservative or Radical?

THE ECHO OF WHAT ONE WOMAN said about endometriosis keeps reverberating: "It is all bound up with the life decisions such as pregnancy and marriage." What was particularly difficult in this woman's case is that she was not married, and there were few prospects on the horizon. She was thirty-five years old and still wanted a family if things could possibly work out that way. She evaluated the options and decided on combined conservative surgery plus follow-up hormone treatment. Radical surgery would have meant removal of the ovaries and therefore no children.

EVALUATING PRIORITIES

Stages III and IV endometriosis are more likely to involve a decision for surgery. The woman in her mid-thirties might be told that she is approaching menopause anyway, so why not have a hysterectomy and get it over with? Somehow this seems like saying we are all going to die sometime, so why not now? Gynecologists often neglect to remind the patient that endometriosis symptoms will be replaced by the symptoms of premature menopause. If the woman has a family she is still raising, these symptoms might be just as disruptive as those of endometriosis.

If conservative surgery is recommended, however, the patient may be faced with recurrence of the condition and future trips to the hospital for more surgery. The continuous chronic pain may take a mental and physical toll as well, not to mention the possible financial burden of medical bills.

If she wants children, she will consider the middle road. In severe cases there is a thin line between conservative and radical surgery. All but a piece of the ovary might be removed.

The decisions about endometriosis are never cut and dried. Endometriosis demands constructive thought and evaluation. Above all, the decisions cannot be reached alone. If a spouse is involved, it is his decision too, along with the doctor, who has an informed opinion.

Some infertile couples hold out for years, with the wife in surgery, on hormones, trying this and that. Finally she chooses radical surgery and a family must be adopted.

One divorced patient found that her boyfriend would have continued their relationship, but he wanted a family in addition to her children by a previous marriage. After years of ineffective treatment for endometriosis, she had to take the path of radical hysterectomy and lose her boyfriend.

Life decisions. They are ours. We must choose carefully the course we take and believe that it is based on sound judgment and concern for all those involved—and most important, for ourselves.

A SECOND AND THIRD OPINION

A woman who lives in Montana, when asked what she would suggest for other women with endometriosis, responded, "At least provide yourself with three different opinions from specialists."

Two would be adequate, if surgery is conservative. But if radical surgery has been prescribed, two additional opinions would be helpful. Radical hysterectomy calls for premeditation and absolute evidence that the surgery is necessary.

Dr. Robert Mendelsohn discusses the growing number of hysterectomies in his controversial book *Mal(e)practice: How Doctors Manipulate Women.* "In the old days," he writes, "a surgeon was the last resort and the patient was referred by the family doctor. Now the patient's gynecologist is often a surgeon, too. S/he not only diagnoses the ailment, but performs the operation."

A case in point: one woman in Boston interviewed for this book recommended that women with endometriosis definitely should find a "good surgeon." Today, about 10 percent of a gynecologist's surgical procedures deal with some aspect of endometriosis, according to W. Gifford-Jones, author of *What Every Woman Should Know About Hysterectomy.* This is a conservative estimate. Other sources go as high as 25 percent.

In teaching hospitals, interns must perform a certain quota of surgical procedures. Women might be advised that hysterectomy is the best alternative, without being told what the other alternatives are. Do not be pushed into any kind of surgery. Tell the doctor that this is a hefty decision that must be given considered time. Be informed. Ask questions, and tell the gynecologist that you want a second opinion.

Insurance companies will pay for second opinions for surgery because they want to be absolutely convinced that the operation they are paying for is necessary. The patient should feel the same way. It might not be coming out of her pocket, but it is coming out of her body.

How does one go about getting a second opinion? Not by referral from the first doctor. Go to another source, a specialist recommended by someone completely unconnected with the first doctor. Women's clinics, hospitals, and medical hot lines often provide referral services. The specialist at another hospital or in another town will not be influenced by previous opinions.

Have your doctor transfer all pertinent medical records and laboratory reports to the second specialist's office. Be sure to explain over the phone while making the appointment that you want a second opinion.

Again, do not lay all your cards on the table. Do not blurt out, "My doctor thinks I need a hysterectomy." Let the second doctor have a chance to formulate an opinion on his or her own.

Some women feel like traitors asking for a second opinion. They are terror stricken to learn that they must have surgery, and most doctors have a talent for intimating "Doctor knows best." Endometriosis is rarely fatal, however, and unless the patient has an ovarian cyst about to rupture or blockage of the bowel by severe endometriosis, there is time. Individual assessment is important. Time may be taken to explore alternatives. Deliberation should be careful, not hasty, especially where castration (removal of the ovaries) is concerned.

If the woman is being hospitalized for laparoscopy, she and her surgeon should agree that if extensive surgery is needed, she will be told about it before it is performed. Smaller implants are often excised during laparoscopy. But if organs are to be removed, the patient has a right to make that decision (unless there is an emergency and her life depends on surgery).

It would be unfair for a woman to go into the hospital for simple diagnostic laparoscopy and come out without her uterus. She should be careful to read all the fine print in any papers she signs upon being admitted and know exactly what the surgeon has in mind. If she is going to have diagnostic laparoscopy and the surgeon wants to scrape or cauterize small implants that might be encountered, she should know of this beforehand.

Usually, the extent of endometriosis will have already been diagnosed when the patient goes into conservative or radical surgery. This is the most reliable order—diagnosis by laparoscopy and biopsy, and then surgery.

HOW CONSERVATIVE?

Where endometriosis is concerned, the word conservative covers a vast territory. Any surgery short of total removal of both ovaries (castration) is considered by many surgeons to be conservative. So the patient who has moderate to severe endometriosis may enter the hospital for conservative surgery and leave without her appendix, with a suspended uterus (see p. 98) and certain nerves cut to relieve pain (see p. 98), a part of one or both ovaries removed, and much more.

Conservative surgery is a catchall term implying that through these procedures the ovaries or a part of the ovaries will be preserved. The lay woman hearing it for the first time might conclude that because her gynecologist has chosen this route, the risk will be less and the procedures simple. To her, conservative means to preserve, within moderate or safe bounds. Surgeons, however, have another concept of the word, especially where endometriosis is concerned.

If conservative surgery is scheduled, the patient should be prepared for one or all of the following:

- excision and/or destruction of endometrial implants
- excision and folding of the uterosacral ligaments in order to suspend the uterus
- appendectomy
- presacral and/or uterosacral neurectomy
- removal by excision of endometriomas on the ovary, and
- possible removal of the uterus, parts of the Fallopian tube(s), and parts of one or both ovaries.

WHAT TO EXPECT

Since the patient will be unconscious on the operating table while all this is going on, perhaps it would be helpful to review the procedures one doctor follows. Dr. S. J. Behrman, at the William Beaumont Hospital in Royal Oak, Michigan, advocated the following procedures at a symposium on endometriosis.

Preoperative Use of Hormones

Behrman finds that combination hormones which effect pseudopregnancy increase the uterus size, make it congested, and soften the implants too much. Some surgeon-specialists such as Dr. Robert Kistner in Boston find danazol which atrophies implants (prescribed for pseudomenopause) more effective in preoperative therapy.

Preoperative Dilation of the Cervix

Behrman widens the cervical opening to reduce the chance of a backflow of endometrial tissue out the Fallopian tubes.

The Incision

Most doctors make the incision in relationship to the severity of the case and the location of the endometriosis. When the endometriosis is severe, Dr. Behrman suggests a midline incision for "optimal visibility." He adds, "The first principle of *all* surgery is visibility," and one "should never use sharp dissection but only blunt separation under direct vision."

Endometriomas

The surgeon must attempt total removal of any endometriomas from the ovaries. Usually this is performed via a wedge resection (taking a piece of the ovary).

Excising Implants

The surgeon will look everywhere, including the posterior peritoneum and the cul-de-sac, for those insidious implants.

Dr. Behrman advises that the surgeon run several feet of the bowel through his or her fingers as well. Sounds tricky and obviously it is. Strict care must be taken not to puncture vital organs.

Cauterizing Implants

Some doctors say yes and others no to cauterizing. Dr. Behrman is firmly against it. He thinks that burn-destroyed tissue has a much greater likelihood of spreading. An exception is made in the case of endometriosis of the cervix. Here, the bluish nodules are usually cauterized.

Suspending the Uterus

Many surgeons routinely perform this procedure, which in more severe cases allows for the raw and tender excised areas in the lower pelvic cavity to heal. One method of surgery holds the uterus in the midline to anterior position for several weeks, giving time to heal. Then the uterus naturally stretches and becomes mobile again.

Appendectomy

In widespread endometriosis, the appendix often is infected, and then there is little question about its removal.

Presacral and Uterosacral Neurectomy

Cutting of certain nerves can reduce pain in the midline area, but not necessarily elsewhere. More about the pros and cons of this controversial procedure will be discussed later (see pp. 99–101).

Postoperative Therapy

The medical profession considers conservative surgery appropriate if the woman desires children. In this case, hormones are usually not indicated, because combined preoperative hormones and conservative surgery should do the job. Incidence of conception is greatest a year subsequent to treatment.

The Ubiquitous Laparoscopy

Most of the surgery for mild to moderate endometriosis will take place by operative endoscopy (surgery using an instrument with its own light source). If the problem area is located in the cul-de-sac (between the back of the uterus and the rectum) and the condition is mild, a culdoscope may be used to remove adhesions through the vagina. In fact, the ovary may be brought into the cul-de-sac area by a special clamp for visualization.

Peritoneal implants may be excised by operative laparoscopy with a midline or suprapubic incision, the same as with diagnostic laparoscopy.

Laparotomy

If the endometriosis is extensive, major pelvic surgery (laparotomy) will be required. An incision is then made in the abdominal wall.

NOTHING IS ROUTINE

Each case of endometriosis is unique. The severity or mildness can be categorized, but until the surgeon actually looks into the pelvic cavity, he or she may only suspect what damage has been done.

Many surgeons who have been taught in medical school to observe certain routine procedures, however, will obey the textbooks to the letter.

Presacral Neurectomy (PSN)

The textbook *Gynecological Endocrinology*, edited by Jay Gold, M.D., and John Josimovich, M.D., states: "Authorities are at odds whether a presacral neurectomy [cutting the nerves in the sacral area of the spine to reduce pain] should be routine. . . . We perform it routinely on all endometriosis patients with dysmenorrhea [pain], retroversion, retroflexion, tubal spasm, or kinking."

As we have noted, painful periods plague a majority of women suffering from endometriosis. If a woman has a moderate to severe case, she can assume (unless told otherwise) that when she undergoes conservative surgery she will be given a PSN.

What are the advantages? Relief from pain would seem to be an obvious advantage, but this is not always the result, especially if the endometriosis has spread to areas not connected with the presacral nerve center.

In addition, the patient must keep in mind that pain is a body mechanism, a warning that something has gone wrong. After the nerves are cut, the endometriosis could be spreading or recurring without pain in the same area without the woman's knowledge.

Uterosacral Neurectomy (USN)

Uterosacral neurectomy is a procedure similar to presacral neurectomy, but the nerves that relay messages from the uterus to the brain are cut. The uterosacral neurectomy prevents spasms of the uterus that may cause a large amount of blood to back up through the Fallopian tubes. Both these routine procedures have serious disadvantages for the woman who has undergone conservative surgery in order to conceive. The pregnant woman who has undergone PSN and USN will not be aware of changes in the first stage of labor. An infertile woman who is having conservative surgery in order to conceive must weigh these consequences. Can she live with the pain until she gets pregnant and the pain disappears? Many women believe that it is better to be numb than to suffer from pain. Some women prefer to be knocked out during their entire adventure of giving birth. But these uterine nerves are indicators in the natural childbirth process. When they are cut and their function denied, the woman may be completely unaware that her time has come to deliver.

Another disadvantage of nerve cutting could be the impairment of normal bowel and bladder function. The patient should seriously consider which is worse, pain or the possibility of incontinence and related problems.

In many areas of the country, if PSN, USN, and uterine suspension are performed as a primary surgical procedure during the laparotomy, the patient will not be reimbursed by Blue Cross and other medical insurance companies. Where the surgery has been conservative, specifically for endometriosis, the chances of reimbursement are much greater. The patient concerned with the financial burden of the operation, however, should investigate ahead of time. She should be aware of what the surgeon plans to do and why. If the word "routine" comes into the conversation, it provides occasion for questioning, especially if the patient has not experienced much pain with her endometriosis.

Appendectomy

A few surgeons feel that since they have the patient on the table, they might as well remove the appendix if the endometriosis has become widespread. They reason that eventually it will have to come out anyway. Preventative medicine, so to speak. Zip and stitch—her appendix will never bother her again (although it may never have bothered her in the first place).

Although an appendix already covered with implants must be taken out, some surgeons seriously question the removal of a perfectly healthy appendix. From contemporary trends in the management of endometriosis, however, it appears that they are in the minority. Some doctors refer to routine neurectomy, uterine suspension, and appendectomy as "The Blue Plate Special."

MICROSURGERY

One woman interviewed during her lunch break from a large university medical center in Massachusetts told the author that she consciously looked for a microsurgeon to perform her second conservative operation for endometriosis because she believed microsurgery was the most likely procedure to preserve the chances of having a family in the future.

In microsurgery, the operating field is magnified by loupes or an operative microscope. All the dissection is done with what is called a Simiens needle using electrocautery. The magnification enhances visualization of implants and minimizes bleeding. Microsurgery is especially useful in ovarian dissection and the excision of penetrating endometriosis.

CONSERVATIVE SURGICAL PROCEDURES
FOR ENDOMETRIOSIS

Uterine suspension: The uterus is suspended to get it out of the way and facilitate healing in the lower abdominal cavity. Often routine.

Presacral and/or uterosacral neurectomy: Nerves are dissected in both regions, especially if there is a history of disabling pain. Often performed routinely.

Appendectomy: The appendix is always examined and might be removed, whether infected or not, as a routine procedure.

Unilateral oophorectomy: One ovary may have to be removed because of an endometrioma that cannot safely be removed.

Resection: Larger lesions are removed surgically. Often a part of the ovary will be dissected (wedge resection) in order to remove an endometrioma.

Cauterization: An electric heat source is used to remove smaller lesions. Effective in the treatment of endometriosis of the cervix.

Hysterectomy: In conservative surgery for endometriosis

this varies, but usually means removal of the uterus. Removal of both ovaries, uterus, and tubes is considered radical surgery.

Myomectomy: Uterine fibroids, which are frequently present with endometriosis, are removed.

Diathermy coagulation: Heat from a high-frequency electrode is used to cut through the tissue of cysts and lesions. This method produces less bleeding.

Suction evacuation: A vacuumlike procedure is used to remove chocolate cysts.

D&C: Some surgeons feel that dilation of the cervix reduces chances of backflow of endometrial tissue out the Fallopian tubes. At the same time the uterus is scraped (curettage) for a biopsy.

Salpingectomy: Excision of a Fallopian tube.

The Laser

Most laser surgery uses a carbon dioxide laser, which emits fifty watts of light as a wavelength of ten micrometers in the infrared spectrum. An ordinary incandescent light bulb emits just about this much light. The difference is that the laser beam is extremely concentrated and can vaporize living cells.

The machine itself is clumsy and expensive (from $20,000 to $50,000). Different instruments, such as flexible optic arms, may be attached. Another accessory that comes with the laser is a vacuum attachment which will vacuum up any leftover tissue, smoke from the laser itself, and other unwanted substances in the field of the operation.

There is one problem: the laser beam is invisible. So a second helium-neon laser, which projects a red beam, is used in conjunction with the carbon dioxide laser. Both pass along the same path, spotlighting the area of surgery.

The laser is widely used in microsurgery, which demands great precision and little bleeding. One of the benefits of the laser is the absence of bleeding. As already mentioned, the cervix is an area where cautery can be performed on endometriosis lesions. The surgeon scans the laser beam back and forth over the area. The laser can cut, seal blood vessels, deaden nerves, and burn away or vaporize diseased tissue.

Some laser surgery may be performed on an outpatient basis. This is similar to spending most of the day in a hospital for a diagnostic laparoscopy without having to pay for expensive overnight accommodations.

HOW RADICAL?

If the surgeon tells the patient that definitive or radical surgery will be required, the case of endometriosis is probably quite severe and extensive. Endometriosis that involves the ovaries and/or bowel is quite serious because of possible rupture of an ovarian endometrioma or obstruction of the bowel.

Dr. Robert Kistner of Harvard said in an interview, "Radical surgery is cancer surgery." We talked about stages III and IV endometriosis, in which every organ is glued to everything else. By cancer surgery he was referring to a radical hysterectomy. Dr. Kistner is a firm believer that the only way to get rid of endometriosis for good is to remove the ovaries (castration).

A woman can have three-quarters of an ovary removed and still retain the capacity to conceive. Whenever possible, surgeons will try to remove the implants by performing what is called a wedge resection, thus saving part of the ovary. But when the patient is older, does not want children, and suffers from disabling pain, the surgeon will most likely suggest complete removal of the ovaries.

A number of surgeons believe that taking out the uterus can eliminate menstrual pain and painful intercourse, although it does not eliminate the endometriosis. Others show a conflict of opinion. The following is a conversation from a roundtable discussion on endometriosis as it appeared in the publication *Patient Care.*

Dr. Berger: Do you remove the ovaries, Dr. Malinak?
Dr. Malinak: Unless the patient is perimenopausal or the ovaries are significantly involved in endometriosis, I try to leave them.
Dr. Marik: I take issue with that! To my mind, the definitive nonconservative treatment of endometriosis includes bilateral oophorectomy [removal of the ovaries].
Dr. Malinak: Well, what about the patient who is thirty to thirty-five?
Dr. Marik: Oophorectomy. We all agree that the growth of endometriosis is promoted by ovarian function.

Whether to leave the ovaries or remove them, that is the question. There are a few good reasons for their removal. In any life-threatening situation, radical surgery will usually be the option. This includes the presence of blood in the peritoneal cavity resulting from a ruptured endometrioma. In this case, the chances of fertility are slim, and eliminating the source of estrogen should diminish the possibility of recurrence. If blockage because of implants threatens the bowel, again, the removal of the estrogen source should inactivate overlooked implants and tissue. An endometrioma on the ovary or ovaries that for some reason cannot be excised will be removed along with the ovary rather than leaving it in with the chance of rupture or malignancy.

Oophorectomy

Surgeons usually allude to the removal of the ovaries as oophorectomy or radical hysterectomy and not as castration. But the physical and psychological implications remain the same. They can be devastating (see below under Hysterectomy). Yet one teacher and artist from Montana found just the opposite to be true. "They performed a total hysterectomy," she confided. "I felt really good and told them I didn't want to take any hormones after the operation. I didn't gain weight or have mustaches—all those things people equate with total hysterectomy and menopause."

Other women are not so fortunate. They must choose between living with the disease or living without their reproductive organs.

Hysterectomy and Early Menopause

All the symptoms concomitant with natural menopause may prevail with menopause resulting from radical hysterectomy: hot flashes, weight gain, growth of facial hair, a feeling of loss, depression, diminished sexual appetite, acne, voice changes, and so on. After the hysterectomy, a great number of surgeons advocate estrogen therapy using drugs such as Premarin that are promoted especially for menopause. They believe that estrogen therapy relieves the side effects of menopause and provides the body with estrogen that was taken away when the ovaries were removed.

Anyone who takes time to think about this will find such logic questionable. It is like taking all the nutrients from flour, bleaching it, and then adding a few nutritional supplements to the white bread. When surgeons prescribe estrogen therapy for the woman who has undergone castration for endometriosis, they are reintroducing the very substance that supposedly caused the endometriosis in the first place.

One doctor who supports castration for extensive endometriosis was asked if the estrogen therapy would cause the endometriosis to return. He reported that there would be little risk of recurrence.

We turn again to Dr. Kistner, whose profession has been devoted to treating endometriosis patients. He writes, "It is rare that the administration of estrogens postoperatively rekindles endometriosis after a hysterectomy and removal of the ovaries."

When asked why a surgeon would put a woman who has had a radical hysterectomy on estrogen, Dr. Paul Manganiello of the Dartmouth-Hitchcock Medical Center said, "We're going on the theory that the surgeon has gotten rid of all the tissue." He cites one case in which he saw a woman who had severe endometriosis and had a radical hysterectomy. She was still young, so the doctors wanted to place her on estrogen therapy to preserve her bone calcium, which falters in post-menopausal women. The woman had another bout of rectal bleeding, however, so they placed her on progestens alone until they were sure the problem had disappeared, then continued on estrogen.

Any woman who elects radical surgery must evaluate and consider these problems. If she does not want to take estrogen, perhaps she should supplement her diet with calcium and inform herself about other supplements that might be beneficial during menopause.

She should also keep in mind that estrogen therapy during and after menopause has been linked with a high incidence of cancer. In *Mal(e)practice*, Dr. Mendelsohn writes, "A number of scientific studies have associated the use of estrogen therapy with an increased incidence of cancer of the breast."

Recurrence Rates

Whether radical surgery or conservative surgery is elected, the woman should continue to see a gynecologist. If she changes gynecologists, it is important to keep the new gynecologist informed of her history of endometriosis.

Recurrence is much greater with conservative surgery. The health book *Womancare* states that the recurrence of endometriosis for "women who don't get pregnant after conservative surgery can be as high as 40 percent."

Figures quoted for complete relief from endometriosis subsequent to total hysterectomy (removal of the ovaries) can run as high as 97 percent, and recurrence rates are low.

9

Radiation Therapy

THE USE OF X-RAYS or radium to remove the ovaries was practiced during the early 1970s. One encyclopedia of nursing
during this time indicates that if surgery is contraindicated,
x-rays in large doses can be applied to destroy the reproductive organs.

Today, Dr. Robert Kistner writes in the textbook *Gynecology and Obstetrics* that at the Boston Hospital for Women
the use of x-rays for nonmalignant conditions has been discontinued. Not only was there a risk of cancer from such
x-ray application, but serious injury could result in the large
and small bowels as well.

If surgery is refused or cannot be undertaken, Depo-
Provera injections can effect menopause and stop ovulation
for at least a year. These injections can also have certain side
effects, but if one must choose between castration by x-ray
or Depo-Provera, it might be concluded that masculinizing
effects and weight gain from the drug are preferable to the
very high risk of cancer.

Dr. George Schneider, Professor of Obstetrics and Gynecology at the Ochsner Clinic of New Orleans, Louisiana,
finds that although x-ray treatment is rare in castration, x-rays

may be used for another purpose. "The surgeon may inadvertently leave behind bits of an ovary," he explains, "because they're difficult to see, or because they're attached to the bowel. When I feel there's any risk of leaving in a remnant, I put in silver clips so cobalt can be aimed at the exact spot to prevent the problem."

Other doctors also practice such therapy for what is called the ovarian-remnant syndrome. From 1,000 to 2,000 rads will usually destroy all traces of overlooked tissue. (An erg is the unit of energy delivered by ionizing radiation; when 100 ergs are deposited in one gram of tissue, the tissue has received one rad.)

In his book on endometriosis published in England almost a decade ago, Dr. J. A. Chalmers makes an interesting observation about radiation therapy and endometriosis. He cites a study on monkeys in which irradiation and endometriosis were linked in a quarter of the recorded cases. He goes on to point out that no such correlation has been established in human subjects, such as in victims of the atomic bomb dropped on Hiroshima. He does not quote directly from any specific study. Endometriosis studies have a tendency to be undertaken in a cursory manner without too much follow-up. One wonders how extensive a study was made of the incidence of endometriosis in the bomb victims.

To show how conflicting the research on endometriosis can be, let us examine an article that was published in *Obstetrics and Gynecology* at about the same time as Chalmers's book. The article summarized a study that centered on women admitted for gynecological problems to two hospitals in Hawaii and one in Japan. The study was conducted on the basis of race. Control groups were white, black, and non-Japanese Oriental women. Researchers found a high incidence of endometriosis in Orientals, and especially in Japanese women.

One must review the figures to understand just how high that incidence was. Of 2,955 gynecologic admissions, 414, or 14 percent, were Japanese; of these women, endometriosis was found in 10 percent. In one hospital 2.8 percent of 1,625 admissions from the white population had endometriosis, whereas 9.2 percent of 87 Japanese patients showed an incidence!

In many ways the study is incomplete, but it does at least make a beginning. In certain respects it produces evidence that brings into question the blanket statement that no correlation has been made between Hiroshima victims and a high incidence of endometriosis. How widespread was radioactive fallout from the bomb dropped on Hiroshima? Did it extend to Hawaii? What is the incidence of endometriosis in the daughters of Hiroshima victims? And why three times the incidence of endometriosis in Japanese women?

Such discrepancies in the literature on endometriosis provoke these questions. The medical literature acknowledges that endometriosis seems to be prevalent in the developed countries. Many researchers have placed the onus of endometriosis on society and the changes that have evolved in the childbearing process and the status of women. But where are the definitive studies on the incidence of endometriosis in American women living in the areas next to the Nevada atomic test sites used for above-ground testing during the 1950s?

A number of surgeons and specialists, considered by other physicians to be controversial, believe that x-ray radiation used for castration actually may cause endometriosis to grow and spread. For many years developed countries have accepted low-level sources of radiation integrated into all phases of high technology, from nuclear power to color TV. The *Handbook on Infertility* published by International Planned Parenthood in 1979 cites radiation as one of the causes of poor sperm quality. Infertility is one of the major symptoms of endometriosis. If radiation can affect the sperm, could not the same be possible in infertile women with endometriosis?

Very few studies have been conducted either to prove or disprove these theories. Intentional x-ray therapy for castration has become passé with the advent of drug treatment and microsurgical endoscopic technology. Nevertheless, conflicting sources have created important unanswered questions about radiation and endometriosis.

10

Rare Complications

Doctors are usually very careful to emphasize that endometriosis is rarely fatal. Such assurance in the age of cancer can be a relief to the worried patient. Endometriosis may be cured. The cure may have unwanted side effects, but unless complications arise, the condition will not be life threatening.

OVARIAN ENDOMETRIOSIS AND OVARIAN CANCER

There are some instances in which carcinoma is found arising in endometriosis of the ovary. These cases are exceptionally rare, but they do occur. One study of ten tumors reported in the medical journal *Cancer* states, "Tumors in the benign, proliferating and malignant categories were often associated with endometriosis in the same or opposite ovary or in another pelvic site."

Another recent study in *Human Pathology* refers to a case of carcinoma arising (from endometriosis) in the wall of the rectosigmoid colon. It was one of the first such cases reported.

Dr. Robert Kistner attests to the uncommon phenomenon. In the chapter on endometriosis from the text *Gynecology and Obstetrics,* he writes, "Only approximately 75 bonafide cases of carcinoma arising in endometriosis have been reported, and a large number of these have been adenoacanthomas. These tumors rarely, if ever, metastasize widely, are rarely fatal, but are prone to local invasion."

Adeno is a prefix meaning glandular; adenocarcinoma is a glandular type of cancer that has been found in the ovary along with endometriomas.

What is the incidence of adenocarcinoma out of all cases of endometriosis of the ovary? One specialist estimates the incidence at 5 percent or less. The transformation of benign endometriosis into cancer can occur in the ovary. But it is rare, and this form of malignancy is usually localized, with a good chance for successful treatment. Only a few cases of endometrioid carcinoma in the rectosigmoid colon have been reported.

ENDOMETRIOSIS OF THE BOWEL

Extensive endometriosis in the bowel can result in blockage, leading to death. Therefore, it is imperative that endometriosis found in the cul-de-sac, on the bowel wall, or in the rectosigmoid area be treated at once. Failure to find the problem can cause progression of the condition, with the ultimate possibility of having to perform a colostomy (surgical procedure to establish an artificial anus) and even of loss of life.

When severe endometriosis in the bowel can be accurately diagnosed, removal of the ovaries to lessen the risk of implants recurring will be advised. Symptoms from endometriosis of the bowel, rectosigmoid colon, and cul-de-sac can include vomiting, painful periods, bleeding from the rectum during menstrual periods, and constipation.

Delay in addressing the problem can lead to serious consequences. Nearly half the cases of peritoneal endometriosis have some sort of intestinal involvement. The bowel adheres to other organs and may be invaded. Unlike cancer, however, the endometrial invasion grows from the outside in, so obstruction is usually one of the last stages of the condition. Early diagnosis and treatment can prevent these late manifestations.

Precise diagnosis and biopsy for possible malignancy are always called for in rectosigmoid endometriosis. Sometimes it is misdiagnosed as sigmoid carcinoma.

ENDOMETRIOSIS OF THE LUNG

More cases of pleuropulmonary endometriosis are being reported. Several specialists interviewed for this book had examined women who had symptoms of spitting blood during their menstrual periods.

Subsequent tests showed the spread of bloody fluid in the lungs, and a diagnosis of endometriosis. Biopsy can be made by inserting a needle (somewhat similar to the process of amniocentesis) into the lungs and withdrawing some of the fluid. It is believed that endometrial tissue found in the lungs has been transported there via the blood/lymph system. Hormone therapy using combination hormones (pseudopregnancy) often produces favorable results.

ENDOMETRIOSIS OF THE NAVEL AND OTHER STRANGE SITES

Tissue from endometriosis has been successfully transplanted to the eyes of monkeys and has grown there. The object was to prove the adaptability of endometriosis and how easily it grows.

In a personal story in *Prevention*, Diane Karnes tells of a lump on her backside. "It became so painful," she recounted, "I couldn't even wear tight underwear. I had the cyst removed. It got worse. After two years, I was told it was not a cyst, but endometriosis."

Another woman questioned by the author in New York had noticed a sore on her navel. A brief time later she was undergoing surgery for endometriosis.

Cases of endometriosis have been reported on the forearm, groin, hand, elbow, and underarm. It is believed that the endometrial tissue in these unusual locations can be explained by the blood/lymph system of dissemination. The inguinal canal is a tubular opening in the lower abdominal wall; in the female it contains the uterine round ligaments (often infected by endometriosis) and the seat of lymph nodes.

As mentioned in an earlier chapter, cases of endometriosis have been discovered in abdominal scars after Caesarian section, hysterectomy, myomectomy (removal of muscle tumor), appendectomy, episiotomy, and also in the perineum (between the vaginal orifice and anus). In these cases, the endometrial tissue is transferred by a needle, a scalpel, or some other instrument used by the surgeon.

SITES OF INCIDENCE

Common

Cul-de-sac (most common)	Posterior wall of vagina
Broad ligaments	Perineum
Uterovesical fold	Ovary (half the cases involve
Rectosigmoid colon	both ovaries)
Appendix	Fallopian tube(s)
Bladder	Rectovaginal septum
Uterosacral area	Bowel wall (exterior)
	Canal of Nuck (round
	ligaments)

Less Common

Ureter	Umbilicus (navel)
Lungs (pleuropulmonary)	Cervix
Inguinal canal (groin)	Vulva
Operative scars	

Rare

Kidney(s)	Thigh
Small intestine	Axilla (armpit)
Elbow	Heart
Forearm	

PART THREE

THE FUTURE

11

Endometriosis in Teenagers

POPULAR MEDICAL LITERATURE on endometriosis sets the average age of women suffering from the disease at approximately twenty-seven to twenty-nine years. But increasing evidence points to a history of endometriosis symptoms in the late teens, and even earlier. Of 365 questionnaires that were sent out and tabulated by the Endometriosis Association of Milwaukee, Wisconsin, a surprising 36 percent of the respondents indicated that they had symptoms by the age of nineteen. Of these, 14 percent were under fifteen.

This is what some of the women with diagnosed endometriosis have written about their early problems.

> I experienced the first symptoms (in my case, very severe cul-de-sac pain when having a bowel movement) when I was nineteen years old. About five years later I began to have the same kind of pain at midcycle and during my periods.

> I have seen a gynecologist since the age of fourteen, always complaining of the same thing, cramps, severe pain, et cetera.

> When I was eighteen, the gynecologist told my mother that everything would be O.K. once I grew up and had a baby.

I had gone through my entire teen years with severe menstrual cramps and discomfort. I was eighteen when a rash of bladder problems broke out.

My doctors have told me there is a chance I might have endometriosis. I am only fifteen years old.

Mary Lou Ballweg and Carolyn Keith, co-founders of the Endometriosis Association, have written the following advice for *Our Bodies, Ourselves:* "We believe that young women with severe menstrual cramps should not be dismissed as experiencing a normal aspect of early womanhood, but should be monitored for possible vulnerability to endometriosis."

THE CAUSE

The retrograde menstruation theory of endometriosis suggests that a backflow of menstrual fluid and tissue is pushed out the Fallopian tubes. This tissue then becomes implanted on the organs in susceptible women. Every month when the woman has her period, the implants also bleed, because they are governed by the same hormones as the uterus. This does not seem a likely explanation, however, for endometriosis appearing in thirteen- and fourteen-year-olds.

Specialists believe that a great many menstrual periods are necessary to cause a buildup of these implants in susceptible women. They find that it takes an average of five years of ovulation for retrograde menstruation to cause endometriosis symptoms.

But endometriosis is thought to proliferate in other ways as well. Endometriosis found in the lungs, for example, could be transmitted there via the blood or lymph system. Various theories for the dissemination of endometriosis also include genetic/familial incidence, hormonal imbalance, and the modification of certain cells outside the uterus.

Drs. Donald Chatman and Anne Ward of the Michael Reese Hospital and Pritzker School of Medicine in Chicago performed laparoscopies on forty-three teenage women who came to them with symptoms of disabling pelvic pain and abnormal bleeding. A high 65 percent of these teenage women turned out to have endometriosis. The average interval between the time these women started to menstruate and the time endometriosis was diagnosed was four-and-a-half years. In older teenage women it is possible that menstrual backup through the Fallopian tubes could have had time to implant.

In cases of young teenagers, researchers such as Dr. Donald Goldstein of the Children's Hospital Medical Center in Boston conclude that this cause is less likely. He suggests that perhaps congenital factors are involved. Genetic/familial connections have been observed in some initial studies. There is a 7 percent tendency for endometriosis to develop in certain families.

Whatever the cause, studies indicate that endometriosis in teenagers is not rare and is being diagnosed with greater frequency.

EARLY DIAGNOSIS AND TREATMENT

Dr. Robert Kistner, who treats patients of all ages for endometriosis, has seen women as young as thirteen years old in his Boston office. "If a girl starts to menstruate when she's nine," he says, "it usually takes five years to develop endometriosis. She can have it when she's thirteen."

The teenager should be aware that untreated endometriosis progresses slowly, but it does progress and is one of the leading causes of infertility today. Delay in addressing the problem can result in childlessness. Early detection and subsequent treatment may help not only to relieve disabling symptoms, but to preserve the chances for childbearing later on.

The Gynecological Exam

The doctor should not disqualify endometriosis, especially if the teenager complains of menstrual pain, lower backaches, and in the case of sexually active teenagers, painful intercourse. These are all symptoms associated with endometriosis. The condition should never be ruled out merely because the patient is young.

What the doctor will want to do is check the reproductive system to determine if there is any blockage or obstruction that might cause a regurgitation of menstrual blood the wrong way into the pelvic cavity, rather than out the body. The gynecologist will also be looking for genital abnormalities such as a retroverted uterus, an imperforate (with no opening) hymen, a double uterus, or a narrow cervix. The physician will try to correct any irregularities.

The Pill and Prostaglandin Inhibitors

Since some doctors believe that retrograde menstruation is the cause of endometriosis no matter what the age, for the treatment of mild cases they will prescribe the Pill in order to simulate pregnancy. Combined hormone therapy suppresses ovulation, causing pseudopregnancy and all but stopping the menstrual flow.

For most doctors, this will be the treatment of choice if the endometriosis has been detected and verified by laparoscopy (looking into the pelvic area via a light-optic scope) and by biopsy. Only if the case is extensive and severe will surgery be recommended for the teenager.

For disabling pain, the doctor might prescribe a prostaglandin inhibitor, even if endometriosis has not been diagnosed. Recently, researchers have discovered that women with severe menstrual cramps (primary dysmenhorrhea) have an excess of hormonelike substances called prostaglandins in their pelvic region, causing extreme spasms of the uterus. A possible link between prostaglandins and endometriosis is now being studied but has yet to be established. The doctor may want to try a drug that inhibits prostaglandins to see if it relieves any symptoms.

Still other doctors will say, "All teenagers have menstrual cramps at the outset," and send the adolescent home with a bottle of painkillers.

A Few Facts

The following statistics were compiled by Dr. Goldstein from a recent study of sixty-six teenage women with diagnosed endometriosis at the Boston Children's Hospital.

- The average age at which the girls started menstruation was 11.8 years.
- The youngest patient was ten-and-a-half years old; her period had started when she was ten.
- Sixty-two percent of the teenagers had pain each month with their periods.
- Thirty-six percent had pain so severe they had to stop normal activities.
- Fifty-six percent were helped by painkillers, the Pill, or prostaglandin inhibitors.
- Twenty-eight percent went to other doctors first (urologists, internists, psychiatrists).
- Twenty-eight percent reported discomfort during sex (but many were reluctant to discuss sexual activity).
- Twenty-one percent reported constipation, diarrhea, vomiting, and nausea with their periods.
- Only 4 percent had severe extensive endometriosis.
- Sixty-five percent showed satisfactory improvement. Others had to stop treatment because of side effects.

Although this is a relatively small study, specialists confirm that they are seeing a greater number of teenagers with endometriosis.

What to Do

Teenagers and parents alike should read as much literature about endometriosis as possible before making an appointment with a gynecologist. The first trip to a gynecologist can be an experience of discovery and wonder for the teenager who has the reassurance of an understanding mother or friend and a careful and sympathetic gynecologist.

Disabling menstrual cramps should always be checked out. Genital abnormalities may often be corrected, solving the problem. If trial treatments such as prostaglandin inhibitors and painkillers do not seem effective, an outpatient laparoscopy and biopsy probably will be performed in order to establish for sure whether endometriosis is involved.

Although the thought of undergoing a gynecological exam may embarrass the young teenager and worry the parent, early detection of endometriosis may prevent future anxiety, heartache, and expense. Treating mild endometriosis in the teenage woman and preserving fertility now will enhance her chances for a normal family of her own.

The Endometriosis Association, established in 1980, is currently forming chapters all over the country and sends out its information packet about endometriosis for a nominal fee. The family doctor may be asked for information about endometriosis or a referral to a gynecologist. If information seems scant, or the doctor expresses skepticism, try to arrange a consultation appointment (just for talking) with a gynecologist specializing in endometriosis. Local women's health centers and hospital medical hotlines ought to be able to refer a perplexed teenager to the right medical source.

Both daughters and mothers should be informed. If the mother or any relatives have had endometriosis, the daughter should be aware that there may be complications with her menstrual periods. If she does not have a close rapport with her mother, the teenager may want to talk to a sister or an older friend. She should not be afraid to ask questions. She might think of this as an important school project that must be well thought out and researched. She can be a health detective for her own body. The relief from pain will be worth this initial investment. So many women who have had severe menstrual cramps and related pain do not take the problem into their own hands until their late twenties, when it is too late.

To Teenagers:

If you think you have endometriosis, speak out. If you feel more natural talking about your body with a woman, look for a woman gynecologist.

True, we all have experienced irregular menstrual periods and some cramping. But if days of school must be missed each month because of too much flow, pain, nausea, and other symptoms, something is wrong.

Find out whether you have endometriosis *now* and avoid minor surgery, chronic progressive pain, irreversible infertility, or even radical surgery later on in your life.

The Endometriosis Association (address: Post Office Box 92187, Milwaukee, Wisconsin 53202) offers an information packet on endometriosis. (See Appendix, p. 182.) They will also send information about membership and about organizing chapters in your area, as well as their newsletter.

12

*Menopause:
Home Free?*

A GREAT NUMBER OF women look upon menopause with
trepidation. They have been led to believe that they will
experience hot flashes, headaches, mood changes, decreased
sexual desire, extra pounds on the scales, and a host of other
annoying signals that their reproductive system is slowing
down.

A woman who has experienced endometriosis on and off all
her life, however, will embrace menopause as the miraculous
cure, the ultimate reprieve from further pain, surgery, medi-
cines, and all the ineffective treatments she may have tried for
many years.

Let us take a look at what some of the consumer literature
has to say about menopause and endometriosis.

- Symptoms certainly improve during pregnancy and
  disappear at the menopause (*Good Housekeeping
  Family Health and Medical Guide*).
- Older women might do well to just sit tight till menopause. The cessation of menstruation and ovulation
  often brings a spontaneous improvement of the condition (Rodale, *Woman's Encyclopedia of Health and
  Natural Healing*).

- Endometriosis also tends to disappear with the onset of menopause (*Ms.* magazine).

Naturally, women would like to believe that endometriosis will go away. But to think that endometriosis will evaporate into thin air when a woman has a baby or reaches menopause is less than realistic.

HORMONES AND MENOPAUSE

What exactly does happen to a woman's reproductive system at menopause? The ovaries stop producing eggs, and levels of progesterone and estrogen diminish. The pituitary gland sends out greatly increased levels of follicle-stimulating hormones (FSH) and lutinizing hormones (LH) to get the system running again. These levels remain quite high for the rest of the woman's life. But for the most part, by the age of fifty or so, the woman's ovarian follicles, which produce the estrogen, have been depleted.

Estrogen

We have already explored the effects of radical surgery, which for our purposes means removal of the ovaries. If surgery is successful, all the remnants of the ovaries will be removed, thus eliminating the primary source of cyclic estrogen in the body. The result will be a premature menopause, and we would hope, a total cure of endometriosis.

We must understand, however, that the ova and follicles are not the only natural sources of estrogen in a woman's body. The adrenal glands also produce estrogen. An androgen (male hormone) produced either by the ovaries, if they remain, or by the adrenal glands is released into the blood. Some of this hormone may be converted into estrone (a type of estrogen) in the fatty deposits of the breasts and the abdomen.

Older women do produce estrogen in this manner, and, in fact, stouter women may undergo a less trying menopausal transition because of a greater amount of this estrogen.

Estrogen Replacement Therapy (ERT)

One woman interviewed for this book had a radical hysterectomy and was sent home with a clean bill of health. Her doctor was firmly convinced that castration meant total cure. He did not even hint that endometriosis could recur.

Fortunately, this woman was smart enough to turn down estrogen replacement therapy (ERT). Her doctor was a proponent of ERT, but she decided that through diet and exercise, she could survive without supplements any concomitant symptoms of premature menopause.

In their book *Women and the Crisis in Sex Hormones*, Barbara and Gideon Seaman write, "Certain supplemental estrogens make endometriosis worse. Some authorities, such as Somers Sturgis, maintain that a history of endometriosis should be a contraindication to ERT. Many physicians do not even ask their patients if they have any such history."

Estrogen can be converted from other hormones in the castrated postmenopausal woman. In fact, in one study of thirty postmenopausal women who retained their ovaries and were being treated for tumors, fourteen were still producing estrogen from their ovaries.

It is evident, then, that the body of the menopausal and postmenopausal woman naturally provides the estrogen it needs. In the patient with endometriosis there is an actual risk in prescribing ERT. Not only does ERT in the older woman increase the risk of cancer, but it can also cause endometriosis to recur.

Few substantial figures exist citing the recurrence rates in postmenopausal women. Here are two observations by leading experts in the field regarding menopause and endometriosis:

Estrogen production, although not cyclic and without additional progestational effect, continues in many patients well past menopause. In such patients, active endometriosis may remain (W. P. Dmowski, M.D.).

There's a certain incidence of recurrence even after bilateral oophorectomy, and there is an incidence of endometriosis in postmenopausal women who are not taking estrogens (L. Russell Malinak, M.D.).

Articles in popular publications continue to intimate, however, that pregnancy and menopause will rid women of endometriosis. In truth, whether menopause is induced or natural, the gynecologist cannot say for sure whether a permanent cure will be the result.

A number of respected gynecologists reassure their patients that bilateral oophorectomy (removal of the ovaries) will put an end to endometriosis problems. Then, the same gynecologists will prescribe noncyclic estrogens to help patients through menopause—noncyclic, because these doctors do admit that cyclic estrogen can cause endometriosis to reactivate. Opponents believe that *any* source of estrogen, either by prescription or from within one's own body, can reactivate endometriosis.

COPING WITH PREMATURE MENOPAUSE

If the endometriosis is extensive, often radical hysterectomy must be performed. But the patient need not be talked into ERT if she is psychologically and physically prepared for menopause. She might want to supplement her diet with vitamins and calcium to curtail osteoporosis (brittle bones), which occurs in most women at menopause. The body has its own source of estrogen from the adrenals, and she must try to enhance her health so that this natural production of estrogen takes over where the ovaries left off. Some women will find that they cannot contend with the "change of life" and will not be able to resist ERT. But remember that menopause is a normal process all women experience. Endometriosis is not.

ADENOMYOSIS

When asked if he treated many older women for endometriosis, Dr. Paul Manganiello, gynecologist at the Dartmouth-Hitchcock Medical Center, said that he did, but they usually were victims of what is known as *endometriosis interna* or adenomyosis. "The uterus is a muscular organ," he explained, "with a shiny lining on the outside, then muscle, then a lining on the inside composed of endometrial glands. *Endometriosis interna* is a condition in which endometrial glands invade the muscle of the uterus."

In other words, the endometrial tissue is still in the wrong place, but instead of gravitating outside the uterus and implanting, it works from within the uterus.

As noted, many physicians tend to lump these two conditions together, although they often seem as different as night and day. *Endometriosis externa* usually occurs in younger women. *Endometriosis interna* is often found in women approaching menopause.

Symptoms

The condition can be accompanied by pain and abnormal menstrual bleeding. Profuse heavy menstrual flow that resembles hemorrhaging is one characteristic of adenomyosis. Some women are symptom-free, and only on examination does the gynecologist observe that the uterus is enlarged and perhaps tender. Pain may be caused if the walls of the uterus become swollen with blood, a condition gynecologists call "boggy uterus." This swelling interferes with the usual elasticity of the muscle structure of the uterus, thus causing pain.

Adenomyosis is extremely difficult to diagnose, short of taking out the uterus, dissecting it, and looking at the tissue under the microscope. Other diseases, such as a certain type of fibroid, may also produce an enlarged uterus and similar symptoms.

The woman with adenomyosis frequently has two or three children. Some researchers believe that a normal weakening of the uterine walls because of childbearing may present a condition favorable to the invasion of the musculature of the uterus by the endometrial tissue.

Unlike *endometriosis externa*, in which the pain may begin before the period and linger afterwards, the pain with adenomyosis is associated with a heavy discomfort during the period itself. Some sufferers of adenomyosis also complain of spot bleeding.

Treatment for Adenomyosis

Whereas *endometriosis externa* often responds favorably to hormonal therapy, adenomyosis does not. In fact, a gynecologist may be able to pinpoint a diagnosis of adenomyosis if the pain worsens with hormone treatment and the uterus seems to enlarge and is even more tender.

Treatment for adenomyosis, therefore, is almost always surgical. Women are primarily in their forties and fifties and have finished their childbearing.

Hysterectomy

One reason gynecologists recommend hysterectomy for adenomyosis is that there is a small risk of malignancy. A few cases of carcinoma arising in adenomyosis have been reported.

Another reason is that, although the woman may be expecting menopause, it may be postponed by the pathological condition of her uterus.

In *endometriosis externa*, a cessation of estrogen production and subsequent menopause will usually cause the external endometrial implants to stop bleeding and regress. But with *endometriosis interna*, the aggravating condition in the uterus may provoke the reproductive system to such an extent that menopause will not take place for several years. In the meanwhile, the uterus can enlarge up to three times its normal size. Constant profuse bleeding during the menstrual period and accompanying pain may convince the patient she cannot wait any longer for menopause to take place.

Externa and Interna: Co-habitants

Whenever a history of external endometriosis affecting the pelvic cavity and region outside the uterus has been established, the gynecologist should also suspect *endometriosis interna*. *These two types of endometriosis exist together in approximately 20 percent of all cases.*

The Older Woman and Endometriosis Externa

Women who are asymptomatic in their younger years can acquire symptoms when they are older. If endometriosis has been progressing undetected for some time, the bowel, colon, and/or ovaries are likely to be involved in the older woman. These areas demand immediate attention. To wait for menopause when endometriosis in these areas is severe presents a great risk.

13

The Career Woman's Disease: Fact or Fantasy?

IN THE FIFTH CENTURY B.C., Hippocrates decided that humans needed to be classified. He devised two types, short and fat (apoplectic) and tall and skinny (phthisic). An updated version of classification stems from the 1940s, when a great deal of classification was being done in Germany and elsewhere. During this time an American psychologist, William Sheldon, decided he would have a go at it. He established three characteristic body types, or somatotypes: the mesomorph, the endomorph, and the ectomorph.

According to Sheldon, these labels were scientifically equated with the layers of cells developing in the embryo. The endoderm predominated in the digestive system; the mesoderm took over in the skeleton and the muscular and circulatory systems; and the ectoderm prevailed in the skin, hair, nails, and nervous system.

Next, being a psychologist, he paired off various temperaments with these somatotypes. When the gut ruled, the *endomorph*, who was fat and round, showed a *visceratonic*, sociable personality. But when the body took command, the *mesomorph*, with a big-boned, athletic body, displayed the *somatotonic* personality, noisy and aggressive. And if the brain dominated, the thin *ectomorph,* with a highly charged nervous system, revealed a *cerebrotonic* personality.

These three classifications for the human anatomy have been widely used in the field of medicine ever since.

SOMATOTYPE

"The endometriosis patient is said to be mesomorphic, caucasian, of a higher socioeconomic stratum, intelligent, overanxious . . ." This statement is quoted from a standard medical text found in medical libraries across the country, *Gynecologic Endocrinology,* edited by Jay Gold, M.D., and John B. Josimovich, M. D.

If we are to believe what is written, the "typical" endometriosis patient (if there is such a patient) is large-boned, with a well-developed, athletic body. But have the authors placed the corresponding temperament in the wrong pigeonhole? According to the popular definition of mesomorph, the woman should be noisy and aggressive. Here, she is called "intelligent" and "overanxious." Do not these characteristics go with the cerebral somatotype?

Classification can be confusing and limiting. Let us take a look at another medical observation appearing in an article on endometriosis in an issue of *Fertility and Sterility.*

> We have observed certain characteristics with sufficient frequency to warrant comment. These women appear to have an intense desire to excel . . . are tense perfectionists with demanding and specific goals . . . [and] are usually well-dressed and have trim figures.

By "trim figures" one would suspect the author is referring to slim women of the ectomorph variety. And yet, the temperament he refers to fits the "aggressive" mesomorph. Could we again be mixing somatotypes?

The following is an excerpt from an interview with specialist Dr. Robert Kistner of the Harvard Medical School:

> [Q] In your earlier articles you talked about a certain type of person with endometriosis. Could you explain this type?
>
> [A] Yes. The mesomorph egocentric. I said that twenty years ago and it's just catching on.
>
> [Q] And you find this is a certain type of woman with endometriosis. Do you mean body structure?
>
> [A] Yes. They're mesomorphic. I've rarely seen a fat woman with endometriosis. It's that type of individual who simply has to clean out the ashtrays all the time.

These comments are from a well-known authority in the field of endometriosis treatment and research. Endometriosis sufferers are defined with a plethora of observations about behavior, psychological makeup, and personality traits. The professionals making the observations are not psychologists or psychiatrists. They do see an inordinate number of women with the condition. They do see women in pain, women anxious to have families, women who have had miscarriages, women who must make decisions about hysterectomies.

When Dr. Robert Kistner, who sees twenty to thirty women with endometriosis a day, says that he has rarely seen a fat woman with the condition, we tend to believe him. When he says that the woman with endometriosis is the type who has to "clean out the ashtrays all the time," we are a little more skeptical.

Most of the above statements from medical texts and interviews are buried in scientific language. They have an aura of authority and thus a ring of authenticity to them. Santa Claus is always round and jolly. Women with endometriosis are always trim and aggressive.

PERSONALITY

It is one thing to say that most women with endometriosis seem to have a certain body build; one can see a person's body build clearly. It is another matter to stereotype the woman with endometriosis as having certain personality traits. The doctor may spend half an hour with the patient three to four times at most before diagnosis and treatment. The patient is often cooped up in a small sterile room, and she has her clothes off.

If the situation were reversed and the gynecologist were sitting on the table waiting for someone to examine his or her tender abdomen and genitals, the reaction might well be overanxious.

Consider another example from the latest edition of the textbook *Gynecology and Obstetrics,* used by medical schools as standard reading for would-be gynecologists: "A specific body type and psychic demeanor are frequently found [in endometriosis patients]. The patient is said to be mesomorphic but underweight, overanxious, intelligent, egocentric, and a perfectionist." Notice that the authors of these textbook chapters write "It is said," or "The patient is said," as if *they* are not saying it. They are just passing on accepted information. But is this information correct? Where are the statistics of patient weights, heights, and bone structures? Are there definitive studies on the patients' intelligence? Why are they called egocentric? Are psychological profiles on each patient available?

Except for statements such as these disguised as holy writ, there is virtually no research by qualified professionals on these gray areas of body type and temperament in endometriosis patients.

When the writers of popular magazine articles and the mass media pass on these statements, then the generalizations and stereotypes hold fast. A recent article on endometriosis that appeared in the *Chicago Sun-Times* and was picked up by the *Los Angeles Times* (circulation 1.1 million) repeats the taglines and labels with gusto.

- It is known as the career woman's disease.
- Childless professional women who are highly motivated and have high-pressure jobs are prone to the disorder.
- Women who tend to have the disorder are usually meticulous in their personal habits.
- Endometriosis is rarely seen in obese or sloppy women.

It is well known that doctors are busy. They work long hours; gynecologists may see up to a score of women in one day. Specialists in a field like endometriosis, where the symptoms can be painful and disabling for the patient, are confronted by a constant barrage of complaints. In writing this book the author became depressed just listening to the stories of women who could not have children because of endometriosis, or who had had up to six operations for the disease, or who were on hormones for months, even years. One can imagine that although this is the doctor's job, it often may not be a pleasant one.

Naturally, the doctor may perceive the patient as anxious and egocentric. She is talking about herself, her pain, her constant problems with this crippling gynecologic condition.

Then there are the women who want to know more about their bodies, who have had enough, who were given ultimatums and not alternatives. They are angry. They have taken the problems into their own hands. Yes, they are aggressive. They have to be. Just one uncaring, unsympathetic doctor can spark a woman to aggression.

Career

One writer and reporter from New Hampshire saw a gynecologist who called endometriosis "the airline stewardess disease." When she asked why, she was told that women who work for the airlines tend to fit the categories: that is, trim, career-minded women who delay childbearing.

What has a career got to do with endometriosis? Dr. John Rock, associate professor of obstetrics and gynecology at the Johns Hopkins Medical Center, thinks that the stressful career has very little to do with the condition. "There are no data to confirm that endometriosis has anything to do with stress," he says. He does correlate late childbearing with endometriosis, however. Many doctors do blame late childbearing for endometriosis, although that correlation is also being questioned because of the high incidence now being detected in teenagers.

Nobody likes to be stereotyped. Granted, if fifty childless stewardesses under thirty years of age, each weighing between 110 and 120 pounds and standing five feet seven inches tall, came to the doctor's office, the doctor might conclude a pattern existed. The doctor, hired by the airline company to treat airline employees, might draw other conclusions as well: that the women were trim, well dressed, and childless.

Another doctor across town who works in a less endowed neighborhood but who has been trained in the diagnostic procedure of laparoscopy might find that his or her endometriosis patients are older teenagers in jeans. That does not necessarily mean that all endometriosis patients are teenagers and wear jeans.

The first doctor might observe that his or her patients have careers. The second will probably say that his or her patients work. Neither statement is representative, documented, or necessarily enlightening.

SOCIOECONOMIC STATUS

Another category that connects with the career label is socioeconomic status. Many doctors believe higher incomes or a high place on the social ladder are characteristics of endometriosis patients. In an interview, one specialist described women with endometriosis. "They're well dressed, usually with a higher socioeconomic level," he said. "A very high percentage are married to lawyers, doctors, bankers, college graduates."

For a doctor to become a specialist involves another investment besides the long years at medical school. Equipment is necessary. The office must be spacious enough to accommodate patients who might travel from all over the world to be treated. Specialists have a high overhead and are expensive, usually too expensive for patients on welfare or of moderate means. As a result, not many tatters and shoes with holes in the soles or patched dresses will be seen in the waiting room of a specialist. People who see specialists can pay, and usually are asked to do so before they leave.

The specialist assumes that these women are financially secure. At least they can pay insurance premiums if they cannot pay the bills themselves. But where are the statistics on the patients who cannot pay at all? They are not in the specialist's office, and so the specialist may assume such women do not have endometriosis.

The question is: Do these women have endometriosis because they have deferred pregnancy, and thus have more periods and more of a chance to build up endometrial implants in their bodies? Or do they have endometriosis because they are married to bankers and lawyers? The question seems absurd, and yet the latter conclusion can be drawn when the two paths of logic are lumped together in this way.

Not very much has been written about our society and the effects of progress, development, and affluence on fertility and other life processes. One contributor in the forefront, Dr. Malcolm Potts, Director of International Fertility Research, explores the subject with vigor. In a recent conversation, he spoke of some of the effects economic growth can have on society.

"In the developing world, the Philippines or somewhere,"

he said, "women reproduce at an early age and there are lots of problems of excess fertility and bringing up the children, which have economic and social consequences, but the women are better off physiologically. The most serious thing, it seems to me, is cancer of the breast, more serious than endometriosis. But they're all diseases related to the postponement of child-bearing."

As more statistics are compiled, we will find out if post-poned childbearing is in fact the cause of endometriosis. At this point, it seems that dealing with the socioeconomic question in relationship to late childbearing is more logical than linking it with career.

Dr. Paul Manganiello approaches the question from the late-childbearing viewpoint too. "Often women [with endo-metriosis] are individuals who have postponed their child-bearing for whatever the reason," he says, "the Korean or Vietnam wars, for example."

There are many reasons for delayed childbearing. The spouse might be sent to war. The couple might want to finish their education. Some women have careers and babies at the same time. Some men and women are ambivalent about having children because they themselves came from unhappy homes. At this point, the variables are too many to come to one conclusion about societal factors and endometriosis.

A NEED FOR STATISTICS

The endometriosis specialist is usually extremely conservative in the diagnosis. He or she wants to see the endometriosis implants via laparoscopy and perform a biopsy before suggesting treatment. This is the scientific method, and it works. Should not the same hold true for the study of somatotype and personality before anyone can write about the "typical patient" in textbooks? If one must describe the "typical patient," is there not a responsibility to qualify, to substantiate and document, to provide exceptions?

Physicians are prone to reporting interesting observations in medical journals. "In my own personal experience, the women I've treated for endometriosis all seem to be trim," the doctor might say. Who is better qualified to note the physical characteristics of the patient than the doctor? This information might appear in an article with some reservations such as "for the most part," "usually it is said," "trends indicate." But, despite these qualifications, mere comment is not clearly distinguished from fact in these prestigious publications.

Does endometriosis relate to the affluence of our society, or even to that of an individual? Nobody can say. In a panel discussion sponsored by *Patient Care*, Dr. Russell Malinak of Baylor College of Medicine in Houston said, "We used to think that the problems of lower socio-economic groups— early pregnancy, tubal blockage due to gonorrhea and PID and so forth—prevented the disease in Blacks. As Blacks and other minority groups climb the socio-economic ladder and defer pregnancy, we see an increased incidence of endometriosis."

In chapter 14 we will take a look at the facts and fantasy surrounding the subject of endometriosis and race. For now, we are concerned with Dr. Malinak's statement for its pairing of socioeconomic status (climbing the economic ladder) and endometriosis. Former statistics concerning a high incidence of endometriosis in private patients versus a high incidence of pelvic inflammatory disease (PID) in ward patients are no longer valid. With the advent of laparoscopy, doctors have conducted certain studies showing the incidence of endometriosis in private (paying) white patients is just about the same as the incidence of endometriosis in black ward (non-paying) patients. How could the researchers before have made such errors? Probably because they learned from their medical textbooks that blacks have PID and whites have endometriosis. So they accumulated the figures but did not have the diagnostic tools or motivation to check them.

It happens that these studies were conducted on the basis of race and not socioeconomic status. But they do point out that ward patients had about the same incidence of endometriosis as private patients. As the techniques for accurate diagnosis become more refined, such myths will probably continue to be destroyed.

Women Start a Data Bank on Endometriosis

Under the supervision of Dr. Karen Lamb, Assistant Professor in the Department of Preventive Medicine of the Medical College of Wisconsin, the data from the first 365 questionnaires sent out by the Endometriosis Association of Milwaukee, Wisconsin, have been computerized. (See Appendix B.) The association has also received a grant from the Winthrop Laboratories (which manufactures danazol) for an independent educational and outreach program. The grant will cover the cost of responses to hundreds of letters sent to the association each week and will help to establish a national media network.

The first questionnaire was eight pages long. Mary Lou Ballweg, co-founder of the association, explains that information was extremely difficult to compile because respondents, glad at last to be able to share their symptoms and problems, wrote lengthy answers. The questionnaire has been revised with an emphasis on shorter answers that are easier for volunteers to tabulate.

The questionnaire asks for age, race, history of symptoms, when symptoms appeared, diagnosis, location of implants, treatments suggested (including pregnancy), what the patient decided to do, result of treatment, recurrence, physician-patient relationships, personal information about tampon use, DES, endometriosis in blood relatives, IUDs, other health problems, tipped uterus, mood, marital status, frequency of intercourse, occupation, education, financial status, and so on.

One part of the questionnaire is called a Time-Line. In it the respondent is asked to state her age at the advent of certain events in her particular history of endometriosis.

Time-Line

Directions: List the age in your life at which the following events occurred. (Please list in order of occurrence.)

Life Events		Example
___first period (menses)	*Age*	*Life Events*
___first symptoms (painful periods)	14	first period (menses)
___first symptoms (pain at ovulation)	16	first symptoms (painful periods)
___first symptoms (pain at other times in menstrual cycle)	19	progesterone (Duphaston)
___first symptoms (painful sex)	20	birth control pills
___first symptoms (infertility)	25	hormone (Envoid)
___definite diagnosis (method of diagnosis _____)	31	diagnosis (laparoscopy)
	31	birth control pills
	32	danazol
Treatments:	32	surgery
___painkillers	33	pregnancy
___anti-inflammatories	34	hysterectomy (uterus and ovaries removed)
___birth control pills		
___danazol		
___progesterone		
___hormones		
___surgery		
___hysterectomy (uterus and ovaries removed)		
___pregnancy or miscarriage		
___use of tampons		
___use of IUD		

A second questionnaire is being revised and reevaluated for programming into the computer data bank. The results will be available to professionals as well as to the association and to women who want answers. Finally, women are joining together to form their own self-help network on endometriosis. Women with babies and continuing endometriosis are not satisfied with the idea that pregnancy cures endometriosis. Teenagers are not satisfied with the cliché that women in their late twenties and early thirties usually have endometriosis. Black women are not satisfied with the suggestion that endometriosis is rare in the black population. Women who work resent the insinuation that career is directly responsible for their condition. Women in pain are tired of being called nervous and overanxious.

They want to find out the truth once and for all. They want to know if prostaglandins, IUDs, tampons, or intercourse during menstruation have anything to do with endometriosis. Women are tired of waiting. They have waited more than a century, and the answers are slow in coming from the medical establishment.

Maybe with the input from hundreds of women from all over the country, patterns will emerge, patterns that could provide, if not the answers, at least long-awaited clues.

THE MAKING OF A MYTH

Robert Mendelsohn, M.D., is a renegade who takes the medical complex and especially the male physician to task. He quotes a statement by the author of *Feminine Forever:* "I seem to detect," writes Dr. Robert Wilson, "a certain look or attitude in some women that one might call 'the birth control look.' Women who have plenty of sex, but no children somehow strike me as vaguely tense and unfulfilled."

Dr. Mendelsohn warns, "The fact that men, as gynecologists are in a position to proclaim these sex stereotypes at any time in the name of *medical science* is an ever-present danger to women."

In the twentieth century doctors pride themselves on being concerned with observation and the classification of facts and establishment of verifiable natural laws. They systematize knowledge that relates to the physical body. But the myth lives on, the heritage of the psychology of the ovary embraced by the nineteenth century. Then, any abnormalities from depression to insanity were attributed to ovarian disease.

At times medical science has a strange way of reversing the adage "seeing is believing." For example, in the nineteenth century, doctors demonstrated that hypersexual urges led to tuberculosis by pointing out the high incidence of the disease in prostitutes.

Today, doctors tell us that they see a high incidence of endometriosis in women with careers. Sometimes they forget to mention that these women delay childbearing, and *that* probably is the physical cause for their endometriosis. And so the myths live on.

14

Race: Turning the Tables

Do WOMEN OF ALL RACES have endometriosis? Until recently, the consensus among doctors has been, no, they do not. Many have said that blacks, Orientals, and Jews are rarely afflicted by the condition. How the doctors arrived at their opinions concerning race and endometriosis remains a mystery.

The *Index Medicus*, which lists articles published in professional journals around the world, shows significantly few entries dealing with the subject of endometriosis in specific races of the United States or elsewhere. Time and again, doctors base their beliefs on the same few outdated articles. Often, the article has been written as many as thirty years ago. Yet most doctors and researchers continue to refer to it and list it as a source.

The state of the art of diagnosis and treatment constantly changes. The same updating should apply to endometriosis. Laparoscopy, the establishment of a wider network of highly trained physicians, and a vast leap in biological knowledge have boosted us far beyond research and studies undertaken in the 1950s, studies that have become obsolete. Perhaps a review of some of the articles available on the study of endometriosis and race will show why.

BLACK WOMEN

That endometriosis is rarely found in black women seems the biggest myth of all. Dr. Herbert Niles, gynecologist and obstetrician in Washington, D.C., says, "That endometriosis has been ignored in the black female is a long-neglected problem."

In a conversation he explained why the neglect probably came about in the first place. Historically, the endometriosis patient was white and private, while ward patients were predominantly black. In those days, in order to diagnose endometriosis, the doctor would have to perform major surgery. So most black ward patients were placed on antibiotics for PID (pelvic inflammatory disease). White private patients were assumed to be of higher economic status and thus able to pay for major diagnostic surgery. The doctor was more likely to take the trouble to perform the necessary surgery for diagnosis in the white private patient.

When asked if there has been a change in the treatment of black women today because of the advent of laparoscopy, Dr. Niles explained, "The problem is that the students listen to what their teachers say as gospel. So when they see a black patient with pelvic pain (even though she has a normal white count, no temperature, no positive cultures), they diagnose her as having salpingitis or PID, rather than doing a laparoscopy to see if she has endometriosis."

Dr. George Schneider of the Ochsner Medical Center in New Orleans observes, "At Howard University College of Medicine in Washington, D.C., they say they are finding a much greater incidence of endometriosis. It's quite likely that years ago black women's symptoms of endometriosis were attributed to PID, and they were treated for that."

Dr. Michelle Harrison, author of the book *A Woman in Residence*, was trained at a teaching hospital known for its policies favoring natural childbirth. It was also one of the better hospitals in terms of responsibility to its patients. But she admits that the black women "rarely get good treatment in the hospital. Even middle-class blacks are treated differently from white women."

Different researchers from the 1950s on have cited the rarity of endometriosis in blacks and among those of poor socioeconomic status. More recently, Drs. C. C. Ekwempu and K. A. Harrison of the obstetrics and gynecology department of a hospital in Zaria, Nigeria, undertook a study of the Hausa/Fulani population. These people live in the Savannah Belt of Nigeria. The population the doctors studied were poor and black. Twenty-seven cases of endometriosis were encountered out of 1,706 major gynecologic operations during a three-and-a-half-year period. In contrast, only seven cases out of 2,976 operations were discovered over a thirteen-year period in female patients of the Forest Belt of Nigeria.

When the statistics are explored, it appears that *endometriosis interna* and *externa* again were lumped together. The Hausa/Fulani women were of menopausal age with associated PID. Almost all of them were of lower economic status. Only two of them had a primary education, and sixteen were unemployed. A high 80 percent had an average of five children.

This particular study raises a number of questions and brings into doubt some "gospel truths" professed by many current textbooks. The Hausa/Fulani are not white, single, childless, and wealthy. Yet they show a high incidence of endometriosis. Their neighbors, who live in the same country with similar economic and racial backgrounds, are relatively free of endometriosis. Why? Could climate be a factor? Inheritance? Religious taboos? Unfortunately, this is as far as the study goes. To the author's knowledge, no subsequent studies concerning these questions have been reported.

Another gynecologist from South Africa also examined the incidence of endometriosis in his black patients. In a recent paper published in the *South African Medical Journal*, Dr. P. F. Venter observes that endometriosis in black patients of Bloemfontein, where he practices, is infrequent. He has not conducted a survey. He has merely observed that the blacks do not have it.

As we have learned, the only way to know whether endometriosis exists for sure is to see the implants and confirm them through a tissue biopsy. Nevertheless, Dr. Venter goes on to say that these women have a high incidence of PID with tubal obstruction, and perhaps that is the reason for the absence of endometriosis. Many doctors believe that tubal obstruction caused by PID prevents the menstrual tissue from backing up through the Fallopian tubes.

One U.S. researcher, Frank P. Lloyd, realizing that most of the studies in the early 1950s had been conducted at large clinics with ward patients, conducted a five-year study at a small community hospital with both white and black private patients. The results showed that the private black patients with the same care as the private white patients showed about the same incidence of endometriosis (7.7 percent in the white patients and 6.9 percent in the black patients).

The Tables Turned

Laparoscopy has turned the tables to a great degree. Drs. Donald Chatman and Anne Ward, who have analyzed data on endometriosis in black teenagers, write, "It has been traditional to view endometriosis as a racially selective illness, rare in Blacks. Although this tenet has been refuted (by Chatman, Lloyd, and others), it still appears in current literature."

The new information has not been assimilated or acknowledged. The myths are being perpetuated. One example appears in the current *Lippincott Manual of Nursing*. The authors advise nursing students that endometriosis "is rarely encountered in women of the Black race." This is only one example of many.

Dr. Herbert Niles, when asked to give the Waldo-Ross Memorial lecture in Washington, D.C., concluded that a more fitting topic could not be found than the discussion of endometriosis. "For the black female," he told the audience, "the realization of the incidence and importance of this condition has been a long time coming." In an interview he said that

Gynecologic Endocrinology, a basic medical text, points to a predilection in the white unmarried private patient. The text adds that endometriosis is "more prevalent in blacks than originally thought."

Dr. Niles expressed his concern as a black physician. "Our own personal experience in recent years with the use of the laparoscope in the diagnosis of unexplained pelvic pain and infertility," he said, "has shown that the incidence of endometriosis in black women is as significant as any other racial group."

> If you are a black woman and your doctor has told you that you have PID, if you are a black woman and have been given antibiotics but your symptoms persist, *act now*. Get a second opinion. Consider having a laparoscopy for a sure diagnosis. You may have endometriosis.

JEWISH WOMEN

The literature that addresses the incidence of endometriosis in Jewish women is extremely scarce. To date, less than a handful of studies have been undertaken.

Dr. A. Brzezinski and his colleagues at the Rothschild-Hadassah University Hospital in Jerusalem published a survey in 1950. Of 1,027 laparotomies, where endometriosis was visualized, they found a low 1.6 percent incidence. This has been one of the lowest percentages in any country studied thus far.

Subsequently, having read reports that the incidence of endometriosis was on the rise in the United States, the Israeli doctors were curious if the same might be true in Israel. So once again they conducted a survey. This time it was more ambitious, covering nearly twenty thousand women hospitalized at the Hadassah Hospital from 1939 to 1961. Of these women, 2,386 had major abdominal surgery. Of these cases (where endometriosis was visualized), *endometriosis externa* was found in only 1.04 percent. This figure is lower than the previous findings. The doctors' results were corroborated by other gynecological departments throughout Israel.

Israel became a state in 1948. Since then, several ethnic and cultural groups migrated to the country, among them many Orientals. Of the twenty-five cases of external endometriosis that the doctors discovered during the twenty-two-year period, only six were in Orientals.

The researchers discussed possible reasons for the low incidence in Israeli women. They believed that genetic factors might be involved. Also, pregnancies were early and frequent in Israeli women. The women observed strict menstrual and marital laws condemning the use of contraceptives and prohibiting sexual intercourse during menstruation. Many of the women wore sanitary pads instead of tampons, believing that menstrual flow should not be hindered.

That was in 1962. Two decades have passed since the study was conducted. Laparoscopy has been introduced. What would the results show now? Israel is not an underdeveloped country. Let us hope that more studies will be forthcoming. If the incidence in Israel remains low, it might provide a clue to this mysterious condition that plagues millions of other women. If, in fact, certain taboos (for whatever reason) improve the quality of health in Israeli women, all women would like to know about it.

Religion and Taboos

Sexual intercourse during the menstrual period is forbidden in Orthodox Judaism. At the end of her menstrual period, the Orthodox Jewish woman takes a ritual bath called a *mikvah*. Only then may she continue sexual relations. The woman is considered unclean during her period. Tampons also are frowned upon.

The Israeli researchers wondered if these taboos, although rigorous (and seemingly sexist to liberated women), might be beneficial in one respect—by reducing menstrual reflux and thus the growth of endometriosis.

Prodded by the plausibility of such conjecture, the author contacted Dr. John Rock, Director of Reproductive Endocrinology at the Johns Hopkins Medical Center. "I know of no study," he said, "that compares the incidence of endometriosis in certain groups of women such as Jewish women who abstain from sex during their periods and women who have intercourse while menstruating."

Once more, we face a dearth of information, despite the fact that endometriosis is a gynecologic crippler that affects an estimated 15 to 25 percent of all women undergoing gynecologic surgery in the United States.

Jewish Patients in New York City

In 1959 two other researchers found a 2.7 percent incidence of external endometriosis in 2,669 laparotomies performed at two predominantly Jewish hospitals in New York City. This is higher than the incidence for Israel, but it is still far below the national average.

As usual, no follow-up studies appear to be available. What is the difference, if any, in the incidence of endometriosis in Orthodox American Jewish women who practice Mosaic laws concerning menstruation compared to American Jewish women who do use tampons and do have occasional sex during menstruation? If no significant difference exists, perhaps the low incidence in the Jewish population is not related to specific taboos at all, but rather to genetic-familial characteristics or childbearing practices. Only by comparisons of this nature will we be able to discern certain patterns. Why some groups of women have endometriosis and others do not must be explored much more carefully and extensively.

ORIENTAL WOMEN

As noted, the non-Oriental communities in Israel showed a higher incidence of endometriosis than the Oriental populations.

Classifiers usually define Orientals as the race east of the Mediterranean with yellowish skin, black hair, and Mongoloid features. Reports in medical journals frequently do not explain what they mean by Orientals but classify peoples as diverse as Japanese, Chinese, and Polynesian all under this general category. Publications or abstracts that report findings on endometriosis among Oriental populations number even fewer than those on black and Jewish women. One study undertaken in 1976 explores the incidence of endometriosis among Japanese women. This study, according to certain standards observed today, might be suspect. It was conducted according to tissue biopsy *or* visualization, not both. Most doctors in the United States feel that one can err on the basis of visualization or biopsy alone. Both visualization and biopsy must be performed for a secure diagnosis.

Other aspects of this particular paper are doubtful as well. In his conclusion the researcher says, "It is generally known that endometriosis is not common among blacks." Several studies even then contradicted such a statement. The researcher does differentiate, however, between *endometriosis externa* and *interna*.

Although inconclusive, the information points to some new patterns. At Tripler Army Medical Center in Honolulu, for example, diverse races were admitted for gynecologic surgery. Of 87 Japanese women admitted, a high 9.2 percent had endometriosis. Non-Japanese Orientals were the second most affected group with an incidence of 5.3 percent. Of the 396 Orientals (Japanese and non-Japanese), the incidence of endometriosis was more than twice that found in Caucasians.

At Kobe Hospital in Japan where admissions were strictly Japanese, of 260 patients, 8.9 percent had endometriosis. This is unusually high for a racial group that has been advertised by doctors as being relatively endometriosis-free.

The Chinese are more than one billion strong. Today, the Chinese practice birth control. It would be meaningless to gather information about endometriosis in China today without knowing what the incidence of endometriosis was in the population prior to the introduction of birth control. Are these statistics available? If, indeed, China's one-child-per-couple program brings about an increase in endometriosis, it could help prove that childbearing and endometriosis are inextricably linked.

We need answers, not theories or isolated studies.

Previously, endometriosis was thought to be rare in black and Oriental women. With the advent of laparoscopy, however, many doctors have discovered that endometriosis is just as pervasive in these races as in Caucasians. Although the latest data are available, for some reason the myth perpetuates in nursing manuals and medical textbooks as well as in popular magazines.

The research field is wide open. But research takes money, effort, and, above all, interest. Nearly one-fifth of all women undergoing gynecologic surgery this year in the United States will have endometriosis. Winthrop Laboratories has established the best-known network in the country for endometriosis research, and concludes, "Endometriosis has been reported to occur in up to 25% of all women in the United States." One out of every four women! About one out of eight women has endometriosis of the ovary. In contrast, it is estimated that one of every hundred thousand women has cancer of the ovary.

Cancer can be life threatening. Endometriosis is not life threatening, but it can cause irreversible infertility. Endometriosis is zero population growth. It threatens future generations. That sounds overly dramatic, but it is true: If allowed to continue undetected, misunderstood, and underfunded, endometriosis could have an effect on our society as profound as any life-threatening disease.

Before it is too late, we must find out why it exists, not just in Caucasians, but in Orientals and blacks as well.

15

Prevention

MANY READERS MIGHT ASK WHY they were not told sooner that endometriosis could be prevented. Actually, the type of prevention we are talking about does not assure immunity or a cure. A better word, and one often used in conjunction with endometriosis, is "management." Unless doctors and their patients know what endometriosis is, how it invades the body, and who it affects, they cannot really prevent it.

For many researchers and gynecologists, the emphasis has been on cure, not prevention. It is easy to prevent a disease when the cause is known. That is what vaccines are all about. There is no vaccine for endometriosis.

There are steps, however, that gynecologists, surgeons, and lay women can take to lessen the chances for the growth of endometriosis. Some of these measures are procedures such as early detection that can minimize the chances of any disease. Others, like nutrition, have been found to work for a few women but are not considered by the medical establishment. Still others, such as therapeutic pregnancy, have been embraced by some physicians but generally are not accepted by their patients.

Endometriosis is already far too widespread to curtail by observing a few simple rules. But the following basic concepts may alleviate widespread endometriosis in the susceptible woman.

EARLY DETECTION

We have reiterated the importance of early detection and diagnosis of endometriosis. One doctor has nicknamed the condition "benign cancer." It travels through the body in much the same ways as cancer, and although it often does not proliferate as fast, women should not procrastinate. Early detection can mean the difference between having a family and not being able to have one. A confirmed early diagnosis, when treated immediately, might even cause the mild case to disappear.

Teenagers especially should be aware of the connection between endometriosis and severe menstrual cramping, lower backache, and other symptoms in connection with the menstrual period. These can be warning signals.

How early is early? As we have seen, one girl with endometriosis seen at the Boston Children's Hospital was ten-and-a-half years old. A number of endometriosis patients start having noticeable problems from their midteens on.

Some women remain symptomless, which makes early detection difficult. Endometriosis may not be diagnosed until a woman wants to become pregnant. If the patient is in her early twenties, the case might still be mild enough to "manage."

Early detection means paying attention to body signals and being aware at puberty of what endometriosis is. Teenagers should be informed about gynecologic procedures and why they must be performed. If teenage girls are old enough to engage in sexual relations by the age of thirteen and fourteen, they must also understand that painful intercourse may not be just the result of their inexperience, but the symptom of a disease.

Early diagnosis depends not only on the teenager but on

her parents and the physician as well. Parents often are reluctant to talk about anything having to do with the reproductive system, including menstruation. Doctors sometimes share this false modesty. Rather than examining the teenager, or sending her to a gynecologist, they will write out a prescription for painkillers.

Reluctance to perform laparoscopy on a teenager is understandable. This is a surgical procedure. If the physician suspects mild endometriosis, the Pill or a prostaglandin inhibitor may serve therapeutically as well as diagnostically on the younger patient.

But the sixteen- or seventeen-year-old with severe pain, backache, constipation, or any number of symptoms associated with menstruation, should definitely be examined by a gynecologist. The gynecologist will then be able to tell if a laparoscopy is in order. We wish more women went into gynecology. Sometimes it is so much easier for a shy, confused teenager to talk with a woman than a man.

CORRECTION OF GENITAL ABNORMALITIES

Some doctors believe that genital abnormalities can lead to endometriosis in susceptible women. Most doctors who discover abnormalities in a young teenage girl believe that such abnormalities should be corrected, if possible, to prevent future problems.

A number of anomalies could cause the backup of menstrual tissue out the Fallopian tubes. The following are a few of the conditions that could provoke endometriosis. Symptoms often arrive at menarche (onset of menstruation) when the blocked menstrual blood starts collecting, causing cramps and, later, painful intercourse.

Cervical stenosis. A congenital narrowing of the cervix. It may be corrected by a D&C (dilation and curettage).

The cervix is expanded with dilators, and the lining of the uterus is scraped clean.

Imperforate anus. Naturally, one could not live with an absence of an opening in the rectum. The condition is corrected at infancy. In one study, however, doctors found that teenage girls who had been treated for imperforate anus as infants later on had a predisposition to endometriosis.

Bicornuate uterus. A double-horned uterus. There is likely to be more bleeding and tissue during periods. Periods often are delayed, and there is sometimes pain with intercourse. The partition between the two horns can be removed. Surgery is usually postponed in a teenager until a major problem arises. Unicorn uterus and other original designs often cause similar complications.

Hematometra. This is a buildup of menstrual blood due to a uterine abnormality and blockage. An incision is made in the hymen. The blood is drained and an antibiotic prescribed.

Imperforate hymen. A thin sheet of membrane completely covers the vaginal opening so that menstrual blood cannot escape. The doctor makes an incision to drain the blood and allow free flow.

Uterine retroversion. When the uterus is tilted backward, doctors usually do not tamper with it in teenagers unless there is a pathological finding or familial predisposition to endometriosis. Approximately one-fourth to one-third of all women have a retroverted uterus.

Stenosis of the hymen. There is only a pinpoint orifice in the hymen; it may be incised to allow free menstrual flow.

Hymeneal occlusion. This is another way of saying that there is a blockage of menstrual blood by the hymen.

Septate vagina. Usually, a double-walled vagina accompanies a double uterus. Surgical removal of the barrier may be performed and an antibiotic prescribed.

Atresia. The partial or total absence of the vagina. It may be treated by plastic surgery so that blood buildup may be drained. An antibiotic is prescribed to prevent infection.

TAMPONS VERSUS SANITARY PADS

Young teenagers who have seen a gynecologist and have been told that they have a narrow vagina, or a small vaginal opening, might be advised to wear sanitary pads instead of tampons. If the menstrual flow is heavy and the opening narrow, it would be healthier to keep that opening as unobstructed as possible. Perhaps with natural growth and the introduction of sexual activity, the opening will dilate and become more elastic.

Since it has been discovered that toxic shock syndrome is caused by bacteria trapped by certain tampon designs, it has been suggested that on lighter days women wear sanitary pads. When the flow is heavier, women should choose the tampon that provides the right absorbency. Tampons have been designed today to gauge and meet specific needs.

So if the teenager wants to use a tampon, perhaps she should select the smaller size. When endometriosis "runs in the family," it might be wiser for her to wear sanitary napkins. She should do all she can to keep the menstrual flow free and unobstructed.

The assumption that tampon use could lead to endometriosis is logical. A tampon is an absorbent plug. If one takes a cotton rag and stuffs it into a drain and then fills the sink, some of the water soaks into the rag, but some of it also fills up in the sink. It seems reasonable to question whether tampons might not work in a similar fashion with menstrual blood.

Dr. Michael Osterholm of the Epidemiology Department of the Minnesota State Department of Health has studied the problem of tampons and toxic shock. In a recent conversation, he said that very little hard data were known to him in regard to tampon use and endometriosis.

Dr. John Rock of the Johns Hopkins Department of Reproductive Endocrinology writes, "The use of tampons is a controversial issue. I don't believe anyone knows the answer."

Dr. Russell Malinak of Baylor College of Medicine in Houston suggests that tampons actually act as a wick, drawing the blood to them rather than blocking it. This theory has been disseminated in popular publications and in tampon advertising, but nothing has been proven one way or the other.

Teenagers should be aware that tampons may compound the problem of a narrow cervix. To be on the safe side, if the adolescent is experiencing disabling menstrual symptoms, she should consider wearing pads to insure freedom of the menstrual flow.

SEXUAL INTERCOURSE DURING MENSTRUATION

If a man shall lie with a woman having her sickness, and shall uncover her nakedness; he hath discovered her fountain, and she hath uncovered the fountain of her blood: and both of them shall be cut off from among their people.
(Leviticus 20:18, KJV)

This menstrual Judaic taboo is as old as Moses (c. 1490 B.C.). Yet very little research on the effects of intercourse during a woman's period has been documented. One Australian researcher conducted a small survey and found that intercourse during menstruation was quite common. In a short but informative letter in the *Medical Journal of Australia*, V. E. Davis addresses this question. He alludes to research by C. A. Fox, in which postorgasmic negative uterine pressure was demonstrated, thus supporting the theory that suction was involved in coitus. Suction pressure could account for retrograde menstruation out the Fallopian tubes during menstrual intercourse.

Let us reread the passage from Leviticus. Could it be metaphorical? In uncovering the fountain of her blood (uterus) during her sickness (menstrual period), both of them could be cut off from their people (made infertile). This is one interpretation briefly explored by V. E. Davis.

Judging from what we know about endometriosis today, the metaphor seems to be in the realm of possibility. (One thirteen-year-old endometriosis patient's history provides an example. She had no genital abnormalities or blockage. She was sexually developed and admitted to frequent intercourse.)

It is popularly thought that at least five years are necessary for endometriosis to establish because of retrograde bleeding due to menstruation. When sex is practiced during menstruation, however, perhaps the penis acts as a plunger, creating suction and causing the movement of amounts of blood and tissue out the Fallopian tubes. In a susceptible teenager, it seems that this reflux might speed up the endometriosis process.

Researchers are still at the hypothetical stage. Dr. Russell Malinak of Baylor Medical College believes that intercourse during menstruation may cause an increase in reflux out the tubes, especially if the uterus is retroverted. But, he adds, "It is unlikely that this fact would significantly influence the development of endometriosis."

In a recent article, Dr. P. F. Venter of South Africa expresses a different opinion. He believes that intercourse and masturbation shortly before, after, or during menstruation may predispose women to endometriosis. Therefore, as a preventive measure, he suggests that women abstain from both during their periods.

In a recent book *From Woman to Woman*, Dr. Lucienne Lanson discusses sex and menstrual cramps. She suggests that orgasm during the menstrual period can help to minimize menstrual cramps. She also points out that if a woman does not have a partner, she may masturbate, thus relieving her cramps. Dr. Lanson recommends wearing a diaphragm when intercourse is performed during menstruation in order to contain the flow. In the endometriosis patient, these suggestions might not be as helpful.

Today, an estimated two-thirds to three-fourths of all women have had intercourse by the age of twenty. One out of four teenagers will get pregnant at least once before that age. Unless teenagers have been educated not to, many of them will undoubtedly experiment with intercourse during their periods. If these teenagers knew that they might be jeopardizing their health and fertility later on, perhaps they might consider abstaining from intercourse during menstruation.

Dr. Fox's initial research indicates that intercourse causes suction within the uterus. A larger study to look into the implications of the practice of intercourse during menstruation is long overdue.

IUD AND CERVICAL CAP WEARERS

Intrauterine devices (IUDs) are notorious for trapping and attracting infection. Studies by pathologist Dr. Nikolas Janovski of the National Naval Medical Center in Bethesda, Maryland, showed that *the IUD will sometimes stimulate endometriosis.*

If a woman suspects that she has endometriosis, she should avoid using the IUD as a means of birth control.

The cervical cap is a contraceptive made of Lucite, rubber, or a similar substance. It fits tightly over the cervix (the neck of the uterus). Cervical caps are not widely prescribed by doctors in the United States. They are much less profitable for U.S. manufacturers than other forms of contraception, so most cervical caps are obtained from abroad.

The cap fits by a suction seal. Recently, a cervical cap with a one-way valve that permits the flow of cervical and menstrual secretions has been introduced. This cap can be left in place during the menstrual period. Long-term studies have not yet been performed.

Could the conventional cervical cap stimulate endometriosis in the same way an IUD seems to? Any answer to that question at this point (and possibly for many years to come) is mere speculation. Doctors do not know for sure what causes endometriosis, nor do they know for sure how the IUD works.

The cervical cap has been around for thousands of years in various guises from molded opium and oiled paper in the Orient to half-squeezed lemons in eighteenth-century Europe. Women find them easy, safe, and comfortable. But since the cap is manufactured chiefly in England, one suspects that research on its use and the incidence of endometriosis (if there is any) will be unavailable for some time to come.

The one-way valve cervical cap worn during menstruation does raise questions. Will the cap permit absolutely free menstrual flow? Or will it promote some menstrual reflux? Dr. Paul Manganiello of the Dartmouth-Hitchcock Medical Center believes that cervical caps might possibly predispose women to endometriosis.

PELVIC STUDIES AND SURGICAL PROCEDURES PERFORMED DURING MENSTRUATION

We have explored the possibility of the spread of endometrial tissue through careless surgical technique. Most doctors advocate precautions to be taken when performing surgical procedures in order to reduce the chances of accidental endometrial tissue transplantation.

- Pumping with a cervical dilator should be avoided, as it can force endometrial tissue out through the Fallopian tubes.
- Any surgical operative procedure should preferably be done *before* the D&C.

- Any surgical procedure involving the cervix and vagina should be avoided before and during menstruation.
- Pelvic examination for endometriosis during menstruation should be *extremely* gentle.
- Postpartum D&C is *contraindicated*, especially on women who have had an episiotomy. Endometrial tissue trapped in the scar can result in endometriosis.
- Endometriosis often appears after electrocauterization. Cautery should be performed three to four days before a woman's menstrual period.
- There is a high incidence of endometriosis associated with scars after a Caesarian. Unless a woman really needs a Caesarian operation, doctors should deliver the baby naturally.
- If a Rubin insufflation test or salpingogram must be performed to find out if the tubes are open, it should *not* be made during menstruation or following a D&C. These procedures can force endometrial tissue out the Fallopian tubes.

In a way, the woman has little control over these procedures. If her gynecologist schedules an insufflation test, however, and does not ask when she expects her next period, she should probably cancel her appointment and look for a more reliable doctor. Or if the pelvic exam is rough and endometriosis is suspected, the woman should try to find someone who is gentle for the following exam. Gentle examination, care, and meticulous surgical technique are imperative for all gynecological work, but especially in the treatment of endometriosis.

BENEFICIAL ASPECTS OF THE PILL

The latest information on the Pill from the Population Information Program at Johns Hopkins University gives it a much better image than it has had in the past. For one thing, the Pill used today is one-tenth the dosage of the original. Women at high risk (over thirty-five who smoke) are also less likely to take it.

The Johns Hopkins report reviews some of the benefits. It announces that there is "documented" proof that "the Pill has a protective effect against cancer of the ovaries and uterus." The report also reduces the concern that the Pill is linked with breast cancer. None of the major studies has discovered such a link. It goes on to indicate that Pill users will have half to one-third less of a risk of developing PID.

The Pill is prescribed for mild to moderate cases of endometriosis. The report does not specify the beneficial or deleterious aspects of oral contraceptives in relationship to the condition. The studies do point to relief from menstrual and premenstrual tension, heavy bleeding, and iron deficiency anemia, however. Let us hope that results on the Pill and endometriosis will be forthcoming.

Dr. Malcolm Potts, Director of the International Fertility Research Program, has been experimenting with new patterns for taking combined oral contraceptives. Traditionally, they have been presented in cyclic twenty-one-day packets. The bleeding that occurs when the woman stops taking the Pill is not normal menstruation but uterine bleeding caused by the withdrawal of hormones.

If a woman wanted, Dr. Potts maintains, she could alter the pattern of this bleeding. He notes that with the "lack of communication between physiologists working on the technical aspects of contraception, and sociologists and marketing experts attempting to increase the acceptance, this element of choice hasn't been exploited previously in nearly twenty years of oral contraceptive use."

Rude awakenings. Again, women have not been informed. The World Health Organization is studying the psychological-social aspects of menstruation. Some women would not feel secure without a monthly period (although with the

Pill it is not really a period). But in several countries, Pill takers have found that they can adapt their so-called periods to fall at a time when they are not working or do not have special engagements.

Dr. van Keep of the International Health Foundation in Geneva has coined the terms "bi-cycle" and "tri-cycle" for the longer-term Pill packages. They are currently being studied in Edinburgh at the Family Planning Association Clinic. Dr. Potts believes that, in physiological terms, extended Pill use is more logical. The Pill simulates pregnancy rather than "normal menstruation."

The study has been advertised and women initially have shown great interest in this new freedom of choice. It is worth noting that endometriosis is often treated with the Pill noncyclically because episodes of uterine bleeding after the twenty-one-day cycles seem to reactivate implants.

Pill use is one area that has been researched extensively. Benefits in relationship to endometriosis have yet to be evaluated, but current studies appear promising.

AN OUNCE OF PREVENTION IS WORTH A SEVEN-POUND BABY

We have discussed the so-called therapeutic baby at great length (pp. 56–58). Naturally, women resent being told to "go have a baby." Doctors deny that they seriously indicate such "treatment." Yet the professional literature continues to emphasize that pregnancy will remediate the condition. Dr. P. F. Venter, under the heading "Prevention" in the *South African Medical Journal*, lists "early marriage and pregnancy without long delays between pregnancies" as important. The prominent medical textbook *Gynecology and Obstetrics* states, "Pregnancy has often been suggested as the optimum prophylactic and therapeutic treatment for endometriosis."

There is little doubt that pregnancy does cause endometriosis to recede. But evidence also exists that recurrence rates are high and that "total cure" is not a sure thing. Also, studies have been conducted in which endometriosis patients had more than one child. In one Nigerian study, the average number of children of the endometriosis patient was five!

Not all the facts are in. Thirteen-year-old teenagers cannot be advised to get pregnant as soon as possible. The old adage, an ounce of prevention is worth a pound of cure, just does not apply in this instance.

To prevent something means to keep it from happening. Pregnancy might place existent endometriosis in check. If the case is mild, it might even cause it to disappear. But the only real reason for having a baby is because a couple wants one.

MENSTRUAL EXTRACTION

The idea of extracting menstrual blood is not new. It was described as "dry cupping" by the obstetrician at Queen Victoria's court. Leeches were thought to serve the same purpose, that is, to draw menstrual blood from the uterus.

The modern form of menstrual extraction was devised by Harvey Karman in 1970. A flexible cannula (tube) was used with a plastic hand syringe to provide the vacuum source.

Today, menstrual extraction is known by many names: menstrual regulation, endometrial aspiration, minisuction, the Karman technique, miniabortion. The procedure is virtually the same.

A cannula is carefully inserted through the cervix and into the uterus. This cannula is fastened to a closed collecting jar that will hold the extracted tissue. A syringe is also fastened to the collection jar. When the syringe is drawn, it creates suction, vacuuming the contents of the uterus through the cannula and into the jar.

The procedure is simple. Dilation and general anesthesia are not necessary. Menstrual extraction is usually performed seven to fourteen days after a woman has missed her period.

There is a distinction between abortion and menstrual extraction. For one thing, the woman often will not be sure she is pregnant. With the introduction of pregnancy tests that may be accurate as little as nine days after a woman has missed her period, the frequency of menstrual extraction has declined.

Certain women's self-help groups perform the procedure on each other. Elton Kessel, in his article "Menstrual Regulation," writes, "This procedure has been advocated by some women's groups in the USA as a matter of convenience to shorten menstrual periods." But two recently published women's health books, *From Woman to Woman* and *Womancare*, advise against menstrual extraction every month. No studies have been conducted to determine the safety of monthly removal of the uterine lining. There is also a risk of perforation and infection, no matter who is performing the extraction.

But let us brainstorm. Suppose that certain new developments still in the future have lessened the likelihood of infection and perforation, so that menstrual regulation every month is harmless. One might then suggest that menstrual regulation would be the perfect prevention for endometriosis. One could remove the endometrial lining and the tissue, and possibly eliminate retrograde bleeding from the Fallopian tubes.

Unfortunately, this is just conjecture. Testing on primates that menstruate and also have endometriosis might lead to information regarding menstrual regulation and its effect on endometriosis.

NUTRITION

A chapter on prevention would not be complete without mentioning nutrition. Yet very little is known about the influence of nutritional patterns on endometriosis.

The Tufts University program on nutrition is one of the most highly developed in the country. An inquiry into current research on endometriosis and its relationship to nutrition, however, yielded virtually nothing. The same applies to several other major universities and colleges with nutrition departments.

One of the few published articles relating nutrition to endometriosis appeared several years ago in Rodale's magazine, *Prevention*. In "How Nutrition Helped My Gynecological Problems," Diane Karnes wrote about her experience with endometriosis. She had undergone two operations and had taken danazol for four months, followed by other hormones. Finally, she decided to follow her own regime.

First, she decided that she should increase the B-complex vitamins, especially choline and inositol. She also increased her protein intake and cut down on sugar. "Although it didn't do much for my endometriosis," she wrote, "I wasn't getting depressed anymore." After a month of this self-prescribed therapy, she went off the hormones. She experienced severe withdrawal symptoms of depression and immediately took two B-vitamin tablets. Within an hour she felt much better. From that day on she tripled her dosage of B vitamins. In the meanwhile, her mother had read that most people are deficient in a mineral called selenium. So Karnes began taking 25 milligrams of selenium a day. Subsequently, she noticed a vast improvement in her endometriosis condition. "I eat as many natural foods as I can," she concluded. "I take a multiple vitamin and mineral tablet in the morning and extra vitamin E, vitamin C, selenium, and B complex at supper. I've never felt better."

Whether this woman cured herself of endometriosis by vitamin and mineral therapy is difficult to say. Judging from the information in her article, she was the victim of careless surgical procedure at childbirth. Her case of endometriosis suddenly appeared as a tender growth on her backside a year after she had her first child.

Karnes does not mention laparoscopy, although one should have been performed to see if the endometriosis was growing in her pelvic area as well. If the endometriosis was transported by surgery and localized in one specific area, it must have been a mild to moderate case (not implicating the bowel or ovaries) and probably would have receded with danazol therapy anyway. Nevertheless, the main point is that Karnes did notice an improvement in her health when she supplemented her diet with vitamins and minerals.

Since doctors often know very little about nutrition, interested endometriosis patients must read on their own and evaluate symptoms in respect to their eating habits. Barbara and Gideon Seaman include a comprehensive chapter called "Vitamins and Minerals That All Women Need" in their book *Women and the Crisis in Sex Hormones*.

The nutrition-conscious woman should be aware that she is treading on unbroken ground when dealing with endometriosis and nutrition. An overdose of vitamins and minerals can be just as harmful to the body as an overdose of any drug. Women should exercise precaution unless backed by sound advice from a professional nutritionist or doctor.

ADDENDUM

Now for the disclaimer. None of these preventive measures will completely eliminate the incidence of endometriosis. But women should be aware that observance of these measures can have a positive effect in curbing it.

16

Leeches and Laudanum:
Grandmother and You

HISTORICAL HIGHLIGHTS

1846   Curette designed by Recamier for scraping the uterus.

1860   Description of endometriosis by Rokitansky.

1873   First systematic study of the condition made by Kundrat.

1860–1921   Only twenty reports on endometriosis found in the literature.

1903   Meyer suggests the "metaplasia theory," in which latent cells are stimulated to change.

1921   Sampson introduces the implantation theory via menstrual reflux.

1922   Sampson coins the word *endometriosis.*

1924   Halban introduces the lymphatic theory, endometrial tissue carried to different parts of the body via the lymph system.

1925   Sampson sees an analogy between endometrial carcinoma and endometriosis.

1952   Fourestier develops the precursor of the laparoscope.

1953 Scott, Te Linde, and Wharton prove that endometriosis may be produced in the laboratory by
transplantation in monkeys.

1968 Laparoscopy is introduced to the United States
and is widely used for diagnosis of endometriosis.

1950–73 Endometriosis is found in approximately 20 percent of all gynecologic laparotomies in the Boston
Hospital for Women.

1975 J. A. Chalmers, M.D., publishes *Endometriosis*,
one of the few medical texts in the English language entirely devoted to endometriosis (currently out of print).

1975 The first large-scale symposium on endometriosis
is organized by Robert Greenblatt, M.D., in Augusta, Georgia.

1976 Danazol, a synthetic derivative of testosterone,
is approved by the U.S. Food and Drug Administration for specific treatment of endometriosis.

1977 Robert W. Kistner, M.D., and colleagues intro-
duce an endometriosis staging classification approved by The American Fertility Society.

1977 Winthrop Laboratories publishes a waiting-room
pamphlet acknowledging that endometriosis occurs in women of all ages and races, mothers and
nonmothers.

1980 The Endometriosis Association is founded by
Mary Lou Ballweg and Carolyn Keith in Milwaukee, Wisconsin.

1981 Terrance Drake, M.D., suggests the use of prostaglandin inhibitors to treat infertility caused by
mild endometriosis.

1982–3 The Endometriosis Association computerizes
365 questionnaires for its new data bank.

1984 The first full-length book on endometriosis is
published for the lay woman.

One lively seventy-three-year-old retired teacher from Michigan talks about her history of endometriosis. "I used to turn over heavy double mattresses when I was twelve," she says, "and I only weighed about ninety pounds. Maybe that's where all the trouble started." By the age of fourteen she had severe cramps. It was 1923 and Lydia Pinkham's tonic was the rage, but, the teacher admits, "It didn't cure anything." A year after she married, she went to the Mayo Clinic, where she was told she had a "webby growth covering her organs and ovaries." She had an operation in which parts of both ovaries were removed. The doctors advised her that if she wanted children she should have them as quickly as possible. At menopause, when she was forty-six years old, she had an endometrial tumor removed. "I've felt better in these later years than I ever did when I was young," she adds. "I always wanted to do things, but it was so hard."

Today, doing things is still difficult for women with severe endometriosis, although now we have learned more about that "webby growth" and have begun to discover alternative treatments.

GREAT-GREAT-GRANDMOTHER

If we think we have problems today, let us consider our great-great-grandmothers.

Madame Veuve Boivin, widowed midwife, and A. Duges, a professor at the Faculty of Medicine at Montepellier in France, wrote a comprehensive treatise titled *Diseases of the Uterus*, which was translated and published in London in 1834. They describe unnatural adhesions of the uterus that cause sterility. The symptoms from these adhesions include "pains and draggings felt in the pelvis, lassitude in the lower limbs, abscesses in the vagina and rectum, and sometimes death." Boivin and Duges give several case histories in their treatise, from which the following are taken. They indicate how "adhesions of the uterus" were treated in the early 1800s.

Madame Kall, twenty-seven years old, "of nervous temperament," caught a lung cold while pregnant in 1826. Twenty leeches were applied; this "was succeeded by abortion and death." Autopsy showed "adhesions of the pleurae," and, the authors continue, "The broad ligaments, the Fallopian tubes, and the ovaria were firmly adherent to the posterior surface of the uterus."

Madame Delam, thirty-two years old, pregnant and of "exceedingly phlegmatic temperament," hemorrhaged. "The uterus was wholly immoveable. Forty leeches were applied without relief; baths, laxative and mild drinks, enemata and opiate liniments were equally unsuccessful. She miscarried and died twenty days later." Autopsy showed the Fallopian tubes and ovaries covered with "adhesions in an inextricable mass charged with pus."

The popular method of treatment for these conditions, in which the "uterus is bound down by its whole circumference," is, according to Boivin and Duges, the application of leeches at the vaginal opening and sometimes at the anus. Baths of sea water or mineral waters are recommended, along with ointments of mercury and specific preparations of gold and balsam. Narcotic injections also seem popular, or a solution of hemlock (let us hope the tree, not the poisonous herb) is introduced into the vagina. A remedy developed from dried autumn crocus seeds is also mentioned. In most of the cases, the "cure" is followed by immediate death. Many of the women described are either sterile or abort in the first or second trimester of pregnancy.

The similarity between the description of these cases as recorded in France in the early 1800s and cases of endometriosis on file in most gynecology offices today is striking.

Boivin and Duges collaborated on this treatise 150 years ago. They note:

a. Rectum turned down to show the adhesions with the uterus.

b. Right Fallopian tube obliterated, and adhering to the ovarium.

c. Left Fallopian tube in a morbid state, adhering to the ovarium.

We know enough about endometriosis to realize that "adherence" and "a bound down uterus" could definitely apply to the condition. These phrases appear regularly throughout this early medical text. The authors also make reference to an earlier description of such "adhesions" by Dr. Weidmann in a book entitled *Memoria Casus Rari* published in 1818.

Currently, the password in the medical community is that endometriosis rarely raised its ugly head prior to the twentieth century. A reading through the nineteenth-century text by Boivin and Duges raises strong doubts about this assumption.

In 1849 the Strong Company of Boston published the "much improved 49th edition" of Dr. Frederick Hollick's *The Diseases of Woman, Their Causes and Cure Familiarly Explained; With Practical Hints for Their Prevention and for the Preservation of Female Health*. In this pocket-size compendium, Dr. Hollick includes a chapter titled "Fixture of the Womb, or Immobility." He explains:

> It frequently happens after an inflammation of the Womb, or adjacent parts, that the *inflamed surfaces* will grow together, so that the different organs will all be united to each other. It is now known that these adhesions are a very frequent cause of Abortion; owing to their preventing the requisite motions of the Womb.

Dr. Hollick continues with the case history of an unfortunate woman who miscarried nine times. He explains that when the adhesions extend to the Fallopian tubes, conception is prevented. As for treatment, the doctor says, "Little assistance can be rendered." He tells of treatment externally with mercurial ointment but warns, "The remedy will not be found generally successful." He does advocate that when a woman has a prolapsed uterus after having a child, inflammation must be subdued to "prevent these adhesions—for certainly little can be done toward curing them." Sound familiar?

Next, he describes the symptoms. "I have known females with adhesions of this kind, who almost constantly felt a dragging at the stomach, as if, to use their own words, everything was going to be torn out of their bodies." Now comes the prophetic passage. "These symptoms," Dr. Hollick continues, "would be relieved by lying down or *by pregnancy* as that elevated the Womb and relieved the strain on other organs." One hundred and thirty years ago, Dr. Hollick recommended pregnancy for an unnamed condition producing adhesions and a fixed uterus. Today, the same recommendation is made for endometriosis.

Dr. Hollick's guide to female health was a best seller in 1849. It had already sold forty-nine editions to women of the day. The lead paragraph of this section points out the commonness of this condition. "It frequently happens," Hollick says. The doctor has not mentioned endometriosis because the word will not be in use until 1922. What Dr. Hollick describes in this chapter could very well be endometriosis. Nevertheless, many contemporary doctors say that endometriosis was extremely rare in the nineteenth and early twentieth centuries and that its incidence has increased only in the last few decades.

Dr. Hollick's "practical hints" are as entertaining as Frankenstein's monster. He describes diseases of the ovary and prescribes "revulsive treatment." This entails implanting horsehair or other annoying substances under the skin to "stimulate" the ovary. After this, hydriodate of potash is rubbed on the skin just above the ovary.

Dr. Hollick's observations and nostrums make fascinating reading. His chapter "Dysmenorrhea, or Painful Menstruate" would be enlightening, and perhaps painfully familiar, to the twentieth-century patient. Hollick's opinions seem to echo those of many present medical school graduates. For example, "Dysmenorrhea is found most frequently in those of a nervous temperament, and in those who are easily susceptible of great excitement."

Later in the same chapter, Dr. Hollick cites the case of a "young lady whose occupation was *teaching* [italics his]. She was intellectual, of a nervous temperament and very industrious, and I have no doubt but that it was her incessant mental occupation that kept up the disease."

The woman had suffered from severe cramps all her life and was ingesting great quantities of laudanum (tincture of opium). She went to Dr. Hollick for galvanism, a popular treatment using electrical currents. But he found that he had to continue the treatment day and night because the pain returned. He did note, however, that galvanism had none of the injurious side effects that heavy doses of laudanum had. He also remarks, "It is probable that if she becomes a mother, the difficulty will disappear." This is a contemporary turn of phrase also.

Hollick's book, as with most of the American medical texts of the nineteenth century, intersperses medical advice with puritan dogma and moral pronouncements throughout. In a section on ovarian diseases, he explains that "the patient is subject to an intense degree of excitement, which sets all self-control at defiance, and leads to moral consequences. *Moral evils* more frequently arise from *physical disease* than many persons suspect." Talking about "Fixture of the Womb," Hollick warns, "Certain vicious and degrading habits in young persons are apt to produce these difficulties."

And so we can see that our great-great-grandmothers not only had to confront endometriosis as a life-threatening disease, but they were forced to carry a heavy burden of moral guilt as well.

GREAT-GRANDMOTHER

Going from puritan America to the age of Queen Victoria does not alter too much for women. In one astounding leap, however, the West does experience electric light, the phonograph, the telegraph, Pasteurization, the typewriter, and a multitude of other inventions.

Meanwhile, doctors still carry around their satchels of homeopathic remedies. The late-nineteenth-century woman might have a new sewing machine, but she still gulps down laudanum for pain. Just one dollar buys ten ounces of the opium tincture. And if she cannot afford the doctor, she does have recourse to mail-order remedies. Female Pills for Weak Women offered by the Sears, Roebuck & Co. catalogue of 1897 are guaranteed to cure all forms of female weakness including "Irregular Periods, Suppression of the Menses, Hysteria, Partial Paralysis, Sciatica, Rheumatism, Swelled Glands, Scrofula," and so on.

Brown's Vegetable Cure for Female Weakness advertises, "Women do not suffer so! Brown's Vegetable Cure will cure you. In all female disorders it is the remedy of the age." Brown's promises to cure nausea, kidney pain, back pain, "bearing down feeling," a dragging sensation in the groin, irregular menses, timid, nervous, and restless feeling, a dread of impending evil, sparks before the eyes, pain in the uterus, hysterics, pain when menses occur, palpitation of the heart, and so on.

Ladies' douches are advertised "for cleansing vaginal passages of all discharges." Hot water bottles are also available for the "weak female." If the doctor does not cure great-grandmother, the marketplace will.

In 1871 W. J. Taylor published *A Physician's Counsels to Woman, in Health and Disease*. This book is more simple and straightforward than the earlier texts. For painful periods due to "displacements of the womb" or the presence of a tumor, Dr. Taylor recommends the following remedies:

- belladonna liniment and glycerin, to be rubbed on the painful area on the lower abdomen
- warm baths
- warm water injected into the vagina

- apiol, an extract of parsley in the form of little pills called "pearls"
- a mixture of camphor, belladonna, sulphate of quinine, and pulverized gum arabic, made into pills
- for those of "idle and luxurious habits," bromide of potassium and water three days before the menses.

The age of science has begun, and Dr. Taylor makes some interesting observations based on studies. He states, "If the wife be fertile, she will have, as an average rule, an infant within the first twenty months of wedded life. If three years pass without the occurrence of pregnancy, the great probability is that she is destined to be barren."

Dr. Taylor candidly points out that this may be the problem either of "the wife or husband." But since his book is for women, he talks about the reasons for sterility in women. He cites a study performed in Edinburgh on "Fecundity, Fertility, and Sterility." Despite a few strange lapses into folklore, Dr. Taylor seems to have latched onto the possibilities of scientific thought. He remarks of these investigations, "These, freed from their sombre statistical array and scientific terminology, we will transfer [translate into everyday language] for the benefit of our non-medical readers." Hallelujah! Dr. Taylor is offering the discoveries of medical research to the lay woman.

The data gleaned from this study is accepted as fact by most gynecologists today. For example: "A woman married between 20–25 years of age is less apt to be sterile than if married earlier or later."

Where the learned doctor seems to jump off the deep end is in discussing solutions for infertility. He notes, "Hippocrates, recognizing the influence of corpulence and leanness upon fertility, advised that thin women should be united in marriage to stout husbands and vice versa."

Dr. Taylor also offers as a matter of observation that "the families of those living among pine trees are usually large. A bed of hemlock boughs, and the odor of pine forests, have both long enjoyed an established reputation in cases of sterility."

Actually, such an ambiance does sound preferable to most twentieth-century infertility clinics.

GRANDMOTHER AND MOTHER

During the next generation women go from wearing clean pieces of sheet or rags during their periods to the riches of manufactured disposable sanitary napkins. In 1915, which is the first year such figures are compiled, sixty-one women die for every ten thousand babies born (as compared to two in ten thousand births today). Emma Goldman and Margaret Sanger start the movement for birth control and contraception while grandmother is still swigging Lydia Pinkham's for her monthly ills. She will flap her way through the 1920s, but every month she will face the same health problems.

Doctors at major clinics now call the webby growth "endometriosis." Surgical techniques rapidly improve with each world war. The risk of surgery is still great, but removing a tumor is possible without immediate death of the patient.

The pessary (a device worn in the vagina) is in use to support the prolapsed uterus and for the retroverted uterus. Laudanum bottles disappear and in the 50s are replaced by tranquilizers. They provide some relief, but endometriosis remains incapacitating. As one grandmother of this era says, "I wanted to do things, but it was just too hard."

YOU

You are lucky. If you have found out that you have endometriosis, you may not feel thankful, but within the last thirty years you have gained the benefits of a highly developed medical technology. If you are infertile because of severe endometriosis, there is more than a 50 percent chance of reversing the situation. Your great-great-grandmother would have lost the child and died herself, never knowing what was wrong with her. She might have been told the pain was because of her "evil ways."

But you know where the condition could come from and possible ways that it implants outside the uterus. Your doctor can actually see it by performing a low-risk diagnostic laparoscopy. In the early eighteenth century the only time the condition was seen was on the autopsy table.

Today, children are not required of you. If you do not want a family, but wish to alleviate a mild case of endometriosis, you may choose combination hormones to simulate pregnancy. Or if you would rather, you may take danazol and effect a pseudomenopausal state in your body.

You have several options. Sometimes, making an informed choice takes a great deal of effort and energy. Great-grandmother had laudanum and Lydia Pinkham's. You have prostaglandin inhibitors, danazol, the Pill, microsurgery, ovarian resection, and, if absolutely necessary, hysterectomy. Great-grandmother had miscarriage, abortion, infant mortality, and possible death in childbirth.

If you are infertile, you have more than a 50 percent chance of reversing the condition and having a healthy baby, and if not, there is laboratory conception, adoption, or a surrogate mother. These prospects may seem glum, but it behooves women to think in retrospect.

Judging from the literature, it is probable endometriosis did exist more than a century ago. Chances are that, as Dr. Hollick says, the condition happened frequently. Whether it occurred as frequently as today we will never know.

A vast difference lies between you and great-great-grandmother. She did what her husband told her. She did what her doctor told her and what society expected of her. Often, she died in the doing. You may do what you choose. Finally, the "life decisions" are yours.

Appendix A

THE FOLLOWING are a few of many organizations that provide women with information about health problems. In addition, most states have women's health clinics and support groups that can offer women with endometriosis understanding as well as pertinent objective data such as referrals to specialists in the area.

Endometriosis Association
P.O. Box 92187
Milwaukee, WI 53203

Founded in 1980, the association already has chapters in several of the larger cities in the country. The Endometriosis Association will send an introductory information packet for $5 (subject to change). Please include a very large (7 × 10) self-addressed stamped envelope with your request. Membership ($15, also subject to change) includes the newsletter. The Endometriosis Association offers support for women with endometriosis, education of the public and medical community about the condition, and promotion of research on the condition. The association provides a newsletter, a data bank, small library, a crisis-call service with trained counselors, speakers on endometriosis for conferences, and so on.

RESOLVE, Inc.
Department R
P.O. Box 474
Belmont, MA

RESOLVE has forty chapters in the United States. It offers a newsletter and information to couples with infertility problems.

The American Fertility Society
1608 13th Avenue S., Suite 101
Birmingham, AL 35205

The society provides a list of fertility centers and specialists located across the country.

Appendix B

THE FOLLOWING are highlights from the Data Bank Report of the computerization and analysis of 365 preliminary questionnaires sent out by the Endometriosis Association. The ongoing study is being undertaken by Dr. Karen Lamb, Professor in the Department of Preventive Medicine of the Medical College of Wisconsin. Since these respondents were self-selected, they are not representative of standard medical surveys. However, the information does lend itself to future studies by other researchers. The enormous response to these questionaires points to a concern by hundreds of women across the United States. Mary Lou Ballweg, co-founder and executive director of the association, highlights some of the more significant findings in the May 1983 newsletter from the Endometriosis Association.

Among the most significant findings in this study of the 365 women is that symptoms of endometriosis (as self-reported by the women) occurred much earlier than the "classic" woman with endometriosis, which medical literature says is in her late 20s and early 30s and is a "career woman." Thirty-six percent of the women in this study reported they experienced their first symptoms before age 20; 14 percent of these in fact experienced their first symptoms before age 15. Another 21 percent experienced their first symptoms before age 25. This is an important finding in relation to diagnosis—doctors need to be alerted to be aware of possible symptoms of endometriosis at a much younger age than previously thought. And education of parents and teens is necessary to make them aware that they should perhaps seek help if problems are occurring and not simply assume young women will "grow out of it." Early diagnosis makes sense particularly in light of the fact that the more this disease has progressed, the harder it can be to treat. In addition, it is important that young girls just coming into womanhood not experience it negatively. This disease, with early onset, could certainly affect a teen's feelings about being a woman and her self-esteem if made to feel the pain or other symptoms were in her head, unimportant, or taboo.

Pain is the most common of all symptoms. Ninety-seven percent of the women in the study experienced pain with their menstrual cycles. What is even more serious is that 62 percent of the women have pain throughout the cycle, not just at the time of menstruation! This is a surprising and very serious finding. What makes this finding even more serious is that *the pain level is characterized by most of the women as severe or moderate, not mild.*

In addition, 59 percent of the women experience painful sex. And 47 percent or nearly half have problems with infertility.

Also significant and interesting was the fact that a large number of women experienced symptoms not traditionally associated with endometriosis in the medical textbooks. Sixty-eight percent reported "diarrhea, painful bowel movements, and intestinal upset" at the time of periods, the most commonly reported symptom after pain associated with the menstrual cycle. (Painful bowel movements have been associated with the disease in the literature in the past—unfortunately, the questionnaire did not list all symptoms separately.) Forty-three percent reported dizziness and headaches at the time of the period or pain. Forty-one percent reported nausea and stomach upset at the time of periods. These symptoms have been linked by other researchers to excessive amounts of prostaglandins (the underlying cause of primary dysmenor-rhea—painful menstruation not due to some other disease). These symptoms, plus the fact that some women with confirmed diagnosis of endometriosis report relief of symptoms with anti-prostaglandins (Motrin, Ponstel, etc.), point to a possible connection between prostaglandins and endometriosis. Perhaps the symptoms are caused by prostaglandins produced by the endometrial implants or by a combination of primary dysmenorrhea and endometriosis in the same woman. It also seems possible that primary dysmenorrhea could cause retro-grade flow of menstrual fluids with its vise-like cramping and set the stage for endometriosis in a susceptible woman. In any case, the data suggests that a trial of anti-prostaglandins might be a useful first treatment and should be perhaps suggested far more often than the data currently shows it is. Another symptom reported by many women which is not usually mentioned in the medical literature was "fatigue, exhaustion, low energy." This symptom was reported by 64 percent of the women.

Another significant study finding was the amount of time the women in the study were unable to work or carry on normal activities due to the symptoms of endometriosis. Sixty-nine percent of the women in the study answered that they had been unable at times to carry on normal work and activities; some stated they felt disabled but had to carry on. The most common amount of time lost was one to two days— 40 percent of the women mentioned that amount of time. One woman answered "3 days every month for 20 years"—which adds up to a total two years lost to pain. Most people would not make light of a disease that took two whole years out of their lives but because the time lost to endometriosis is often periodic (in every sense of the word!), others do sometimes tend to make light of it. Too many women have stated (on questionnaires and elsewhere) that they've lost jobs or had to go to part-time work because of absences due to endometriosis.

Finally, of great interest were the findings on danazol, about which the Association receives more questions than about anything else related to endometriosis. *One hundred and eighty women in the study had taken danazol or were taking it at the time of the study for a total of 1009 months (or 84 years) of use.* One hundred and sixty of these women responded to the question of whether the danazol relieved the symptoms of endometriosis. Fifty-one percent of these said danazol relieved symptoms; 23 percent said it offered some relief or relieved the symptoms temporarily. Nine percent said it was too early to tell; 12 percent said they obtained no relief of symptoms. A surprising finding was that some women reported no relief while on the drug.

One hundred and forty-six of the women provided information on the recurrence of endometriosis following danazol therapy. Of these, 55 percent said the endometriosis had recurred; 22 percent said it had not; and 23 percent said they did not know or it was too early to tell. A flaw in the questionnaire was that it did not ask how long the woman had been off the danazol. Most of the questionnaires in this study were completed in late 1980 and in 1981 when the drug had only been used widely a couple years—thus, it is possible that the recurrence rate is underrepresented here since most of the women had not been off the drug for very long. As with other treatments, the study did not correlate extent of disease with treatment results or dosage or length of time on the drug with results for individuals.

All the women reported side effects with danazol. The most common were weight gain—73 percent; water retention and bloating, 53 percent; depression and irritability, 53 percent; menopausal-type symptoms, e.g., hot flushes or dry vaginal lining, 53 percent; masculinization symptoms—51 percent. In addition, 71 of the 180 wrote in other side effects they had experienced.

Glossary

ADENOMYOSIS   Condition in which the endometrial lining of the uterus invades the muscular wall. Also known as *endometriosis interna.*

ADHESION   Fibrous band of tissue that binds organs or parts of them together.

ADNEXAL   "Are close to." Organs that are close to others.

AMENORRHEA   Absence of menstruation for a prolonged time.

AMNIOCENTESIS   A diagnostic procedure in which fluid is drawn from the amniotic sac in pregnant women to determine the sex and condition of the fetus.

ANABOLIC   A chemical substance that causes synthesis of body proteins. Danazol, used in the treatment of endometriosis, is an anabolic.

ANDROGEN   Male sex hormones that have a masculinizing effect in females. Danazol is an androgen.

ANOVULATION   Failure to ovulate.

ANOVULATORY BLEEDING   Uterine bleeding that has not been preceded by ovulation.

ANTIGEN   A substance that stimulates the production of antibodies.

ANTIBODIES   Specific substances produced in the blood that react to antigens. A part of the body's defense mechanism.

ARTRESIA   Closing of a normal opening.

AUTOIMMUNE RESPONSE   Reaction against a substance, often a protein, of the patient's own body.

BASAL BODY TEMPERATURE   The lowest body temperature recorded just on waking. Variations can determine when a woman is ovulating and thus is optimum for conception.

BENIGN. Nonmalignant.

BSO   Bilateral salpingo-oophorectomy, surgical removal of the Fallopian tube and ovary on each side.

BIOPSY   Excision of tissue for microscopic examination to establish a diagnosis.

CANNULA   A hollow tube for withdrawal of fluid from the body.

CASTRATION   In the female, removal of the ovaries.

CAUTERIZATION   The destruction of tissue, usually with a laser; used to treat endometriosis of the cervix.

CERVICAL STENOSIS   Narrowing of the cervix.

CHOCOLATE CYST   A saclike structure formed from endometrial tissue and filled with "tarry" blood.

COITUS   Sexual intercourse.

COLPOSCOPY   A binocularlike instrument used to detect abnormalities of the cervix and the vagina and to take a tissue sample for biopsy. This is performed as an office procedure.

COMBINED HORMONES   A pill with both estrogen and progesten used for contraception and for the treatment of endometriosis.

CONIZATION   Removal of a cone-shaped part of the cervix by knife or cautery.

CORPUS LUTEUM   The yellow body formed in the ovary after rupture of a follicle and release of the ovum. Present in ovulation. Absence of corpus luteum indicates an anovular cycle often associated with endometriosis.

CUL-DE-SAC   Fold of peritoneum forming a pouch between the uterus and the rectum.

CURETTE   A spoonlike instrument used to scrape the uterus.

DANAZOL   An antigonadotropin that suppresses the release of

FSH and LH from the pituitary. Used to produce pseudo-menopause in endometriosis patients.

DANOCRINE   Trade name of danazol, produced by Winthrop Laboratories for the treatment of endometriosis.

D&C   Dilation and curettage. The cervix is dilated and the uterus scraped with a curette. This procedure is often indicated for *endometriosis interna.*

DYSMENORRHEA   Painful menstruation. Primary dysmenorrhea is painful menstruation with no known organic cause.

DYSPAREUNIA   Difficult or painful intercourse.

ECTOMORPHIC   Predominance of structures from the ectodermal layer of the embryo, developing skin, nerves, sense organs, and brain, and developing the slender body build.

ECTOPIC   Extraordinary site.

ENDOMETRIAL   Referring to tissue that lines the inner walls of the uterus.

ENDOMETRIOMA   A chocolate cyst; a tumor of tissue from the endometrium.

ENDOMETRIUM   The mucous lining of the inner uterine wall.

ENDOMETRIOSIS EXTERNA   Presence of endometrium outside of the uterus in ectopic sites.

ENDOMETRIOSIS INTERNA   Adenomyosis; a benign invasion of the endometrium into the uterine wall.

ENDOMORPHIC   Predominance of structures developed from the endodermal layer of the embryo, developing the internal organs and producing a corpulent body build.

ENDOSCOPE   An instrument of the fiber-optic type permitting photography and biopsy. The light fibers travel a flexible tube.

EPISIOTOMY   Incision made in the perineum (area between vagina and anus) during the birth of a child when the vaginal orifice does not stretch enough.

ESTROGEN   A hormone produced mainly in the ovaries. When the ovaries are removed, small amounts are produced by the adrenal glands in women.

FALLOPIAN TUBES   Two tubes that open out from the upper part of the uterus. They convey the ova into the uterus.

FIBROIDS   Benign tumors that are found in the uterus. They can be imbedded in the inner wall. They often occur along with endometriosis.

FIXED UTERUS   The uterus is "frozen" into one position. In severe endometriosis it is often bound in this way.

FSH   Follicle-stimulating hormone, a hormone from the pituitary that stimulates the growth of ovarian follicles (sacs containing the ovum).

GONADOTROPIN   Any hormone that stimulates the male or female sex glands. FSH and LH are gonadotropins.

HEMATURIA   Blood in the urine.

HYMEN   A thin mucous membrane across the lower opening of the vagina.

HYSTERECTOMY   Surgical removal of the uterus and cervix. The extent of the surgery and definition varies with the doctor.

HYSTEROSALPINGOGRAM   A test with contrast x-rays taken while dye is injected into the uterus to determine on a corresponding screen if the Fallopian tubes or uterus are blocked.

HUHNER TEST   Cervical mucous is examined immediately after intercourse when the woman is ovulating to determine if the sperm were able to penetrate the mucous and survive.

IMMUNOLOGY   The study of the body's own defense mechanisms against certain diseases that invade the body.

IMPERFORATE HYMEN   A fold of mucous membrane at the vaginal entrance with no natural outlet for menstrual fluid.

INFERTILITY   Inability to conceive or have children.

INGUINAL CANAL   Tubular opening in the lower abdominal wall containing uterine round ligaments.

INGUINAL NODE   A lymph node in the groin and a site of endometriosis.

INTRAUTERINE Within the uterus.

LAPAROSCOPY A diagnostic procedure using an endoscope (light-optic source) inserted just below the navel to observe the pelvic cavity and reproductive organs. Performed with biopsy for diagnosis of endometriosis; also used surgically.

LEUKOCYTOSIS Increase of white cells in the blood. Endometriosis may produce a higher white cell count.

LH Lutinizing hormone, one of the pituitary hormones that influence ovulation.

LYMPHATIC SYSTEM A complex of vessels that drain off and filter tissue fluid. Nodes for this drainage are located throughout the body; it is thought that endometriosis can spread using this system.

MENARCHE Age at which a woman's menstrual periods begin.

MENOPAUSE Cessation of menstruation permanently. It may be caused prematurely by removal of the ovaries.

MENORRHAGIA Excessive menstrual flow.

MENSTRUATION The flow of blood and endometrial tissue from the uterus and out the vagina that occurs about once a month in women in order to prepare the uterus for possible pregnancy.

MENSTRUAL EXTRACTION Withdrawal of the contents of the uterus with a flexible tube called a cannula. Also known as endometrial aspiration, minisuction, the Karman technique, menstrual regulation.

MESOMORPHIC Predominance of structures from the mesodermal layer of the embryo, developing bone, muscle, and connective tissue, and producing an athletic body build.

METASTASIS Transference of disease from one part of the body to another.

METORRHAGIA Spot bleeding between periods.

MICROSURGERY Small-scale surgery performed with loupes or magnifying lenses and often with the aid of a laser and laparoscope.

MULTIPARA A woman who has had more than one child.

NODULE   A small firm lump or mass, which can be malignant or benign. Nodules can be palpated (felt) by doctors during the course of a pelvic exam. Some endometrial cysts and tumors are referred to as nodules.

NOSOCOMIAL DISEASE   A disease incurred in a hospital or clinic through careless procedure or surgical technique.

OSTEOPOROSIS   Loss of bone density due to progressive calcium deficiency. The disease occurs mostly in menopausal or postmenopausal women with low estrogen levels.

OVARIAN WEDGE RESECTION   Removal of a part of the ovary or ovaries.

OVARY   Female sex gland.

OVULATION   The maturation and rupture of follicle (sac), releasing the ovum (egg).

OVUM   The egg produced by the ovaries (plural *ova*).

PATENT   In reference to the Fallopian tubes, unblocked.

PID   Pelvic inflammatory disease. Any inflammation and/or infection of the female reproductive system.

PERINEUM   The area between the anus and opening to the vagina.

POSTPARTUM   Occurring after a baby is born.

POUCH OF DOUGLAS   Recto-uterine cul-de-sac, or dead end.

PRESACRAL NEURECTOMY   Routine cutting of the nerves in the uterine area to reduce future pain. This procedure is often routine in endometriosis patients.

PRIMARY INFERTILITY   Inability to conceive and reproduce.

PROGESTEN (PROGESTIN)   Progesterone. This form of the name sometimes refers to the synthetic hormone.

PROGESTERONE   A hormone produced by the corpus luteum.

PROPHYLAXIS   Prevention.

PROSTAGLANDINS   Hormone-amino acidlike substances found in large amounts in women with menstrual cramps and women with endometriosis. They cause smooth muscles of the uterus to contract.

PROSTAGLANDIN INHIBITORS   Drugs that suppress prostaglandins.

PSEUDOMENOPAUSE   The continuous use of a male hormone (androgen) to lower the body's hormone levels and simulate a state of menopause.

PSEUDOPREGNANCY   A simulated state of pregnancy brought on mainly by progesten-based oral contraceptives prescribed on a continuous basis for six to nine months.

PYELOGRAPHY   Radiographic visualization of the renal pelvis and ureter by injection of a radiopaque liquid. Used to detect endometriosis of the ureter.

PYURIA   Pus in the urine.

RAD   A measure of radiation. A rad equals the absorption of 100 ergs of energy to one gram of body tissue.

RADICAL HYSTERECTOMY   Usually, this mean surgical removal of the uterus, Fallopian tubes, and ovaries.

REFLUX   The backup of menstrual tissue through the Fallopian tubes and outside the uterus. Also referred to as retrograde menstruation.

RENOGRAM   Diagnosis of kidney disease by x-rays following injection of an opaque medium.

RETROVERTED UTERUS   A tilting backward of the entire uterus so that the cervix points forward. Found in a number of patients with severe endometriosis.

RUBIN INSUFFLATION TEST   Carbon dioxide gas or air is blown through a tube into the uterine area to determine if the Fallopian tubes are free and open.

SALPINGITIS ISTHMICA NODOSA   A disease presenting nodular lesions in the Fallopian tubes. Frequently mistaken for endometriosis and vice versa.

SECONDARY INFERTILITY   Inability to conceive after having had one or more children.

SOMATOTYPE   Body build of an individual.

SONOGRAM   A record made by applying sound waves to the female reproductive organs. Sonography can be used in endometriosis to detect tumors of the ovaries.

STROMA   The foundation of the chocolate cyst or endometrioma; the part that bleeds is the stroma.

THORACENTESIS Inserting a hollow needle into the pleural cavity (of the lungs) to draw out fluid for biopsy.

TAH Total abdominal hysterectomy. The body of the uterus and the cervix are surgically removed.

TROCAR A pointed rod that fits inside a fiberglass sleeve; used in laparoscopy.

UMBILICUS The navel.

URETER Tube that drains urine from the kidneys.

URETHRA Channel leading from the bladder to outside the body.

ULTRASOUND High-frequency sound waves are targeted at the body via a microphonelike device. The waves bounce back in echo patterns to form a picture on a screen. Sometimes used to detect tumors of the ovary.

UTERINE SUSPENSION Routine surgical procedure performed on endometriosis patients (stages III and IV) to draw the uterus up to a midline position for healing purposes.

Bibliographical Notes

THE MAJOR reference sources are listed in the order they appear in the text of each chapter. The subject of the reference is set off in italics beneath the entry. In some cases, this notation applies to a general subject introduced in the chapter and not to a specific statistic or quote.

PART ONE/THE CONDITION

1 *Endometriosis: Women and Life Decisions*

ROGER SHORT, "Future Developments in Fertility Control," in *Birth Control: An International Assessment*, ed. Malcolm Potts and Pouru Bhiwandiwala (Baltimore: Park Press, 1979), pp. 215–25.

healthy women in society

LYNDA MADARAS and JANE PATTERSON, "The Menstrual Cycle in the Mature Woman," in *Womancare* (New York: Avon, 1981), pp. 61–73.

explaining menstruation

Good Housekeeping Family Health and Medical Guide (New York: The Hearst Corp., 1979), p. 87.

explaining endometriosis

ROBERT B. GREENBLATT, *Recent Advances in Endometriosis*, International Congress Serial no. 368, a symposium held in Augusta, Ga., 1975. (New York: Elsevier, 1976), Foreword, p. vii.

after fibroids, endometriosis is commonest

2 *The Endometrium and Endometriosis*

ROBERT W. KISTNER, "Endometriosis as a Cause of Infertility," in *Progress in Infertility*, ed. S. J. Behrman and Robert W. Kistner (Boston: Little, Brown & Co., 1975), pp. 345–63.

Sampson coined word

J. A. SAMPSON, "Peritoneal Endometriosis Due to the Menstrual Dissemination of Endometrial Tissue into the Peritoneal Cavity," *American Journal of Obstetrics and Gynecology* 14 (1927), p. 422.

retrograde menstruation

J. A. SAMPSON, "Intestinal Adenomas of Endometrial Type," *Archives of Surgery, London* 5(1922), pp. 217–80.

Sampson's theories

BARBARA VARRO, (*Chicago Sun-Times*) "Endometriosis the 'Career Woman's Disease' of Uterus." *Los Angeles Times*, 25 March 1982.

all women have retrograde menstruation, not just a few

R. B. SCOTT, R. W. TE LINDE, and L. R. WHARTON, JR., "Further Studies on Experimental Endometriosis," *American Journal of Obstetrics and Gynecology* 66(1953), p. 1082.

studies with monkeys

J. A. CHALMERS, "Aetiology and Histogenesis of Endometriosis," in *Endometriosis* (London & Boston: Butterworths, 1975), pp. 6–11.

obstruction of menstrual flow

ROBERT B. GREENBLATT, "Endometriosis: The Nature of the Problem," in *Recent Advances in Endometriosis*, International Congress Serial no. 368, a symposium held in Augusta, Ga., 1975 (New York: Elsevier, 1976), p. 9.

muscle spasms as cause

Patient Care. "Endometriosis: New Views, New Therapies," round-table discussion in *Patient Care*, 12, no. 19 (Darien, Conn.: 15 November 1978), p. 27.

third-degree retroverted uterus

ROBERT W. KISTNER, "Endometriosis" (prophylaxis), in *Gynecology and Obstetrics*, ed. John Sciarra (Hagerstown, Md.: Harper & Row, 1980), chap. 38, p. 24, reprint.

third degree retroverted uterus

CARL T. JAVERT, "Pathogenesis of Endometriosis," *Cancer*, No. 2 (May 1949), pp. 399–408.

metastatic lymph theory

J. A. SAMPSON, "Inguinal Endometriosis," *American Journal of Obstetrics and Gynecology* 10(1925), p. 462.

lymph theory

ROBERT S. MENDELSOHN, *Mal(e)practice: How Doctors Manipulate Women* (Chicago: Contemporary Books, 1981), p. 84.

nosocomial disease

A. KAUNITZ and P. A. DI SANT AGNESE, "Needle Tract Endometriosis," *Obstetrical Gynecology* 54(1979), pp. 753–55.

in amniocentesis scars

"Endometriosis: New Views, New Therapies," round-table discussion in *Patient Care* (Darien, Conn.: 15 November 1978), p. 27.

immunologic link

ROBERT COOK, "Reconnoitering the Body's Main Line of Defense," *Boston Globe*, 18 July 1982, p. 71.

immunology

L. Russell Malinak et al., "Heritable Aspects of Endometriosis," *American Journal of Obstetrics and Gynecology* 137(1980), p. 335 (discussion by Dr. George T. Schneider).
immunology

J. A. Sampson, "Heterotopic or Misplaced Endometrial Tissue," *American Journal of Obstetrics and Gynecology* 664(1925), pp. 730–38.
cancer and

Kathryn Schrotenboer and Genell J. Subak-Sharpe, "The Menstrual Cycle," in *Freedom from Menstrual Cramps* (New York: Pocket Books, 1981), pp. 21–23, 29–32.
hormones defined; prostaglandins

Robert B. Greenblatt, *Recent Advances in Endometriosis*, a symposium held in Augusta, Ga., 1975 (New York: Elsevier, March 1976), Foreword, p. vii.
benign cancer

Abraham E. Rakoff, "Differential Diagnosis Between Endometriosis and Other Conditions Causing Pain and Dysmenorrhea," in *Recent Advances in Endometriosis*, symposium held in Augusta, Ga. (Elsevier, March 1976), pp. 14–15.
adenomyosis

C. C. Ekwempu and K. A. Harrison, "Endometriosis Among the Hausa/Fulani Population of Nigeria," *Tropical and Geographical Medicine* 31(1979), pp. 201–5.
researchers dividing into interna and externa camps

Joe Simpson et al., "Heritable Aspects of Endometriosis," *American Journal of Obstetrics and Gynecology* 137(1980), pp. 327–31.
endometriosis as a general term

3   *More a Condition Than a Disease*

Good Housekeeping Family Health and Medical Guide (New York: The Hearst Corp., 1979), p. 87.
definition

LYNDA MADARAS and JANE PATTERSON, *Womancare* (New York: Avon, 1981), p. 373.

definition

DAVID R. ZIMMERMAN, "En-do-me-trĭ-ōsis," *Ladies Home Journal*, March 1975, p. 54.

definition

PAMELA JANE GRAY, "Endometriosis: The Career Woman's Disease?" *Ms.*, January 1981, p. 74.

15 percent of all women

MADARAS and PATTERSON, "Cancer," in *Womancare*, pp. 661–93.

cancer; routes of dissemination

JOHN C. WEED and PIERRE C. ARQUEMBOURG, "Endometriosis: Can It Produce an Autoimmune Response Resulting in Infertility?" *Clinical Obstetrics and Gynecology* 23(1980), pp. 885–93.

immunology

"Endometriosis: New Views, New Therapies," round-table discussion in *Patient Care* (Darien, Conn.: 15 November 1978), p. 27.

immunology

MADARAS and PATTERSON, *Womancare*, p. 421.

80 percent of women with endometrial cancer
have history of menstrual irregularities

JOE SIMPSON et al., "Heritable Aspects of Endometriosis," *American Journal of Obstetrics and Gynecology* 137(1980), p. 327.

incidence in families

JOE SIMPSON et al., "Heritable Aspects of Endometriosis. I. Genetic Studies," *American Journal of Obstetrics and Gynecology* 137(1980), pp. 327–31.

incidence in families

L. RUSSELL MALINAK et al., "Heritable Aspects of Endometriosis. II. Clinical Characteristics of Familial Endometriosis," *American Journal of Obstetrics and Gynecology* 137(1980), pp. 332–37.

incidence in families

4 *Symptoms*

ROBERT W. KISTNER, "Endometriosis as a Cause of Infertility," in *Progress in Infertility* (Boston: Little, Brown & Co., 1975), pp. 345–63.

30 percent asymptomatic

KATHRYN SCHROTENBOER and GENELL J. SUBAK-SHARPE, "Symptoms of Endometriosis," in *Freedom from Menstrual Cramps* (New York: Pocket Books, 1981), p. 77.

asymptomatic

ARTHUR FRANK and STUART FRANK, "Endometriosis," *Mademoiselle*, February 1978, p. 174.

symptoms

ROBERT B. GREENBLATT and ISMET SIPAHIOGLU, "Endometriosis: The Nature of the Problem," in *Recent Advances in Endometriosis*, International Congress Serial no. 368, a symposium held in Augusta, Ga. (New York: Elsevier, 1976), p. 9.

dysmenorrhea

"Endometriosis: New Views, New Therapies," round-table discussion in *Patient Care*, 12, no. 19 (Darien, Conn.: 15 November 1978), p. 38.

pain and psychological overlay

ROBERT W. KISTNER, "Endometriosis," in *Gynecology and Obstetrics*, ed. John Sciarra (Hagerstown, Md.: Harper & Row, 1980), chap. 38, p. 20, reprint.

every implant menstruates

Ibid., p. 22.

pelvic exam during menses

Winthrop Laboratories, New York. "Endometriosis" (1978), p. 5.

25 to 40 percent of infertile women

J. A. CHALMERS, *Endometriosis* (London & Boston: Butterworths, 1975).

> *symptoms according to site*

ABRAHAM E. RAKOFF, "Differential Diagnosis Between Endometriosis and Other Conditions Causing Pelvic Pain and Dysmenorrhea," in *Recent Advances in Endometriosis*, International Congress Serial no. 368, symposium held in Augusta, Ga. (New York: Elsevier, 1976), pp. 12–16.

> *adenomyosis; salpingitis; hernia; PID*

ROBERT W. KISTNER, "Endometriosis As a Cause of Infertility," in *Progress in Infertility* (Boston: Little, Brown & Co., 1975), pp. 345–63.

> *appendix affected in 9 percent*

ROBERT W. KISTNER, "Endometriosis" (differential diagnosis), in *Gynecology and Obstetrics*, ed. John Sciarra, (Hagerstown, Md.: Harper & Row, 1980), chap. 38, p. 22, reprint.

> *other diseases similar to*

L. IFFY, "Outcome of Pregnancy Subsequent to Induced Abortion," *American Journal of Obstetrics and Gynecology* 138 (1980), pp. 587–88.

> *pregnancy and*

L. IFFY, "Experimental Design for the Surgical Relocation of the Ovary," *International Journal of Fertility* 24(1979), pp. 270–75.

> *ectopic pregnancy*

LYNDA MADARAS and JANE PATTERSON, "Gonorrhea," in *Womancare* (New York: Avon Books, 1981), pp. 543–48.

> *diagnosing*

5 Infertility: A Major Symptom

LYNDA MADARAS and JANE PATTERSON, "Gonorrhea," in *Womancare* (New York: Avon Books, 1981), p. 622.

> *definition of infertility; 30 percent lower male sperm*

CAROL POGASH, "This Story Has a Happy Ending," *Redbook*, August 1982, pp. 81–86.

infertility and

"Endometriosis: New Views, New Therapies," round-table discussion in *Patient Care*, 12, no. 19 (Darien, Conn.: 15 November 1978), p. 37.

ovulation and

Linacre Laboratories, New York. "How to Use Your Ovulindex Thermometer," 1974.

fertility and basal body temperature

LUCIENNE LANSON, "To Have: How to Become Pregnant," in *From Woman to Woman* (New York: Knopf, 1980), chap. 16, pp. 235–36.

Rubin test; Huhner test

The American Fertility Society, "Classification of Endometriosis" (adopted in 1978).

classification and staging

ROBERT W. KISTNER, "Endometriosis as a Cause of Infertility," in *Progress in Infertility*, ed. S. J. Behrman and R. W. Kistner (Boston: Little, Brown & Co., 1975).

studies on infertile women

KATHRYN SCHROTENBOER and GENELL J. SUBAK-SHARPE, in *Freedom from Menstrual Cramps* (New York: Pocket Books, 1981), pp. 33–49.

prostaglandins

"Prostaglandins, Culprits in Cramps, Are Tied to Endometriosis-Infertility," *Medical World News*, 11 May 1981, p. 41.

prostaglandins

DIANE KARNES, "How Nutrition Helped My Gynecological Problems," *Prevention*, August 1979, p. 116.

therapeutic baby

PART TWO/TREATMENTS

6 *Laparoscopy and Other Methods for Diagnosis*

ROBERT W. KISTNER, "Endometriosis" (observation and analgesia), in *Gynecology and Obstetrics*, ed. John Sciarra (Hagerstown, Md.: Harper & Row, 1980), p. 24, reprint.

expectant treatment

KATHRYN SCHROTENBOER and GENELL J. SUBAK-SHARPE, *Freedom from Menstrual Cramps* (New York: Pocket Books, 1980), p. 37.

80 percent respond to prostaglandin inhibitors

ARTHUR FRANK and STUART FRANK, "Endometriosis," *Mademoiselle*, February 1978, p. 174.

painkillers; waiting

LYNDA MADARAS and JANE PATTERSON, "Endometriosis" (diagnosis), in *Womancare* (New York: Avon, 1981), p. 378.

risks of waiting

JOHN E. GUNNING, "The History of Laparoscopy," in *Gynecological Laparoscopy*, ed. Jordan Phillips and Louis Keith (New York & London: Stratton Intercontinental Medical Book Corp., 1974), pp. 62–65.

laparoscopy, history

J. A. CHALMERS, "Diagnosis of Endometriosis," in *Endometriosis* (London & Boston: Butterworths, 1975), p. 25.

suggests against culdoscopy
if endometriosis is in cul-de-sac

J. PHILLIPS et al., "Laparoscopic Procedures: A National Survey for 1975," *Journal of Reproductive Medicine* 18(1977): pp. 219–26.

risk of laparoscopy

"Endometriosis: New Views, New Therapies," round-table discussion in *Patient Care*, 12, no. 19 (Darien, Conn.: 15 November 1978), p. 72.

cost of laparoscopy

F. JAROSLAV HULKA, "Sterilization by Laparoscopy," information booklet published by The American College of Obstetricians and Gynecologists.

outpatient laparoscopy

MICHELLE HARRISON, *A Woman in Residence* (New York: Random House, 1982).

laparoscopy

Good Housekeeping Family Health and Medical Guide (New York: The Hearst Corp., 1979), p. 773.

laparoscopy, description

Department of Nursing, Mary Hitchcock Memorial Hospital, Hanover, N.H., "Diagnostic Laparoscopy Information Sheet" and "D&C Information Sheet."

before and after laparoscopy

J. A. CHALMERS, "Histological Appearances," in *Endometriosis*, 1975, pp. 18–19.

description of cysts

W. P. DMOWSKI, "Current Concepts in the Management of Endometriosis," *Obstetrics and Gynecology Annual*, 1981. Ed. Ralph Wynn (E. Norwalk, Conn.: Appleton Century Croft, 1981), vol. 10, p. 281.

description of cysts

DAVID R. ZIMMERMAN, "En-do-me-trĭ-ōsis," *Ladies Home Journal*, March 1975, p. 54.

description of cysts

MADARAS and PATTERSON, *Womancare* (New York: Avon, 1981), pp. 375–76.

60 percent of all endometriosis cases involve ovaries

Ibid., pp. 748–49. *ultrasound, general description*

ROBERT S. MENDELSOHN, *Mal(e)practice: How Doctors Manipulate Women* (Chicago: Contemporary Books, 1981), p. 164.

risks of ultrasound to lab animals

M. DELAND et al., "Ultrasonography in the Diagnosis of Tumors of the Ovary," *Surgery, Gynecology and Obstetrics* 148 (1979), pp. 346–48.

distinguishes benign from malignant tumors

ANDREW HOPKINS et al., "Pelvic Endometriosis as Demonstrated by Gray Scale Ultrasound," *Journal of the National Medical Association* 71 #3(1979), pp. 289–90.

ultrasound, nonspecific diagnosis

SERGE DALLEMENT et al., "Endometriosis with Uretic Involvement: Preoperative Sonographic Evaluation," *New York State Journal of Medicine*, 79 #3(1979), p. 383.

ultrasound, nonspecific diagnosis

7 Medical Treatment

LUCIENNE LANSON, "To Have Not: How to Avoid Pregnancy," in *From Woman to Woman* (New York: Knopf, 1981), p. 253.

25 different combined hormones

HAROLD SILVERMAN and SIMON GILBERT, *The Pill Book* (New York: Bantam, 1979), p. 230.

oral contraceptives

BARBARA SEAMAN and GIDEON SEAMAN, *Women and the Crisis in Sex Hormones* (New York: Bantam, 1977), p. 136.

vitamin therapy for pill users

"Endometriosis: New Views, New Therapies," round-table discussion in *Patient Care*, 12, no. 19 (Darien, Conn.: 15 November 1978), p. 79.

hormones not advised

"Endometriosis: Continuing Conundrum," editorial in *British Medical Journal*, 281 (1980), p. 889.

how hormones work

Endometriosis Association, "Danazol and the Treatment of Endometriosis" (Information Series #1).

danazol

Winthrop Laboratories, New York: "Endometriosis," 1978, p. 10.
combination hormones and danazol

VEASY C. BUTTRAM et al., "Interim Report of a Study of Danazol for the Treatment of Endometriosis," *Fertility and Sterility* 37 #4(1982), p. 481.
side effects of danazol

BARBARA SEAMAN and GIDEON SEAMAN, *Women and the Crisis in Sex Hormones* (New York: Bantam, 1977), p. 503.
irreversible side effects of danazol

"Endometriosis: Continuing Conundrum," editorial in *British Medical Journal*, 281(1980), p. 889.
danazol partially effective

Postgraduate Medical Journal (supplement on danazol) 55, #5 (1979).
pregnancy and danazol

L. RONNBERG et al., "Effects of Danazol in the Treatment of Severe Endometriosis," *Postgraduate Medical Journal* 55 #5 (1979), p. 21.
relief from pain with danazol

"Endometriosis: New Views, New Therapies," round-table discussion in *Patient Care*, 12, no. 19 (Darien, Conn.: 15 November 1978), p. 6.
recurrence with danazol

W. P. DMOWSKI, "Current Concepts in the Management of Endometriosis," in *Obstetrics and Gynecology Annual*, ed. Ralph Wynn (1981), vol. 10, p. 301.
recurrence with hormones

8 Surgery: Conservative or Radical?

ROBERT S. MENDELSOHN, *Mal(e)practice: How Doctors Manipulate Women* (Chicago: Contemporary Books, 1981), p. 83.
surgeons

W. GIFFORD-JONES, *What Every Woman Should Know About Hysterectomy* (New York: Funk & Wagnalls, 1977), p. 26.
endometriosis 10 percent of gynecological surgery

S. J. BEHRMAN, "Surgical Management of Endometriosis," in *Recent Advances in Endometriosis*, International Congress Serial no. 368 Symposium held in Augusta, Ga. (New York: Elsevier, 1976), pp. 60–66.
surgery and

JAY GOLD and JOHN B. JOSIMOVICH, "Endometriosis," in *Gynecologic Endocrinology* (Hagerstown, Md.: Harper & Row, 1980), p. 435.
surgery and

MARY HAMMOND and LUTHER TALBERT, *Infertility* (University of North Carolina Health Sciences Consortium, 1981), p. 93.
bladder and bowel problems with neurectomy

JEFF HECHT and DICK TERESI, "Laser Medicine: A Bright Promise," in *Laser* (New Haven, Conn.: Ticknor & Fields, 1982), pp. 67–68.
the laser and surgery

"Endometriosis: New Views, New Therapies," round-table discussion in *Patient Care*, 12, no. 19 (Darien, Conn.: 15 November 1978), p. 90.
radical surgery

LYNDA MADARAS and JANE PATTERSON, "Endometriosis," in *Womancare* (New York: Avon, 1981), p. 326.
recurrence with conservative surgery

9 Radiation Therapy

ROBERT KISTNER, "Endometriosis," in *Gynecology and Obstetrics*, ed. John Sciarra (Hagerstown, Md.: Harper & Row, 1980), p. 42, reprint.

"Endometriosis: New Views, New Therapies," round-table discussion in *Patient Care*, 12, no. 19 (Darien, Conn.: 15 November 1978), p. 96.
radiation and ovarian remnants

J. A. CHALMERS, "Radiation," *Endometriosis* (London & Boston: Butterworths, 1975), pp. 56–58.

radiation and the atomic bomb

KUNIO MIYAZAWA, "Incidence of Endometriosis Among Japanese Women," *Obstetrics and Gynecology*, 48 (1976), pp. 408–8.

high incidence in Japanese women

International Planned Parenthood, *Handbook on Infertility* (London: 1979), p. 14.

infertility and radiation

JOHN W. GOFMAN, *Radiation and Human Health* (San Francisco: Sierra Club Books, 1981), pp. 760–853.

radiation and Hiroshima-Nagasaki victims

10 Rare Complications

LAWRENCE ROTH et al., "Ovarian Endometrioid Adenofibromatous and Cystadenofibromatous Tumors," in *Cancer*, 48 (1981), pp. 1838–45.

cancer

SHIGERU AMANO et al., "Endometrioid Carcinoma Arising From Endometriosis of the Sigmoid Colon" in *Human Pathology*, 12 (1981), p. 845.

cancer

ROBERT W. KISTNER, "Endometriosis," in *Obstetrics and Gynecology*, ed. John Sciarra (Hagerstown, Md.: Harper & Row, 1980), pp. 16–17, reprint.

cancer and

"Endometriosis: New Views, New Therapies," round-table discussion in *Patient Care*, 12, no. 19 (Darien, Conn.: 15 November 1978), p. 52.

carcinoma and endometriosis of the ovary

ROBERT W. KISTNER, "Endometriosis," p. 10.

half of the cases intestinal

DIANE KARNES, "How Nutrition Helped My Gynecological Problems," *Prevention*, August 1975, pp. 114–15.

ectopic sites

PART THREE/THE FUTURE

11   *Endometriosis in Teenagers*

DONALD GOLDSTEIN et al., "Adolescent Endometriosis," *Journal of Adolescent Health Care*, 1(1980), pp. 37–41.

in teenagers

DONALD CHATMAN and ANNE B. WARD, "Endometriosis in Adolescents," *The Journal of Reproductive Medicine*, 27 #3 (1982), pp. 156–60.

in teenagers

BARRY SCHIFRIN et al., "Teen-age Endometriosis," *American Journal of Obstetrics and Gynecology*, vol. 116 #7(1973), pp. 973–80.

in teenagers

12   *Menopause: Home Free?*

W. P. DMOWSKI, "Current Concepts in the Management of Endometriosis," *Obstetrics and Gynecology Annual: 1981*, ed. Ralph Wynn (Appleton Century Croft, E. Norwalk, Conn.: 1981), vol. 10, p. 285.

menopause and estrogen

LUCIENNE LANSON, *From Woman to Woman* (New York: Knopf, 1981), p. 332.

estrone, self-produced estrogen

BARBARA SEAMAN and GIDEON SEAMAN, *Women and the Crisis in Sex Hormones* (New York: Bantam, 1979), p. 399.

estrogen, ERT, and contraindication in endometriosis

A. E. RAKOFF, "Differential Diagnosis Between Endometriosis and Other Conditions," in *Recent Advances in Endometriosis*, symposium held in Augusta, Ga.: 1975 (New York: Elsevier, 1976), p. 15.

20 percent of adenomyosis cases exist with endometriosis externa

"Endometriosis: New Views, New Therapies," round-table discussion in *Patient Care*, 12, no. 19 (Darien, Conn.: 15 November 1978), p. 90.

estrogen and menopause

13 *The Career Woman's Disease: Fact or Fantasy?*

The Body (Alexandria, Va.: Time-Life Books, 1964), pp. 40–41.

classifications of somatotype

PAMELA JANE GRAY, "Endometriosis: The Career Woman's Disease?" *Ms.*, January 1981, p. 74.

Dr. John Rock; stress; no data to link with endometriosis

VEASY C. BUTTRAM, "Conservative Surgery for Endometriosis in the Infertile Female," *Fertility and Sterility*, 31 (1979), p. 118.

personality and somatotype

BARBARA VARRO, *Chicago Sun Times*, "Endometriosis the 'Career Woman's Disease' of Uterus," *Los Angeles Times*, 25 March 1982.

personality traits

ROBERT W. KISTNER, "Endometriosis," in *Gynecology and Obstetrics*, ed. John Sciarra (Hagerstown, Md.: Harper & Row, 1980), pp. 17–18, reprint.

personality and

"Endometriosis: New Views, New Therapies," round-table discussion in *Patient Care*, 12, no. 19 (Darien, Conn.: 15 November 1978), p. 28.

socioeconomic connection; wealth and

Endometriosis Association, *Newsletter*, September 1982, p. 1.

computer data bank for

ROBERT S. MENDELSOHN, *Mal(e)practice: How Doctors Manipulate Women* (Chicago: Contemporary Books, 1981), p. 98.

sex stereotypes

BARBARA EHRENREICH and DEIRDRE ENGLISH, *Complaints and Disorders: The Sexual Politics of Sickness.* Glass Mountain Pamphlet #2. (Old Westbury, N.Y.: The Feminist Press, 1973), p. 30.

> ovarian rule of temperament; sexual activity and TB

14 Race: Turning the Tables

"Endometriosis: New Views, New Therapies," round-table discussion in *Patient Care*, 12, no. 19 (Darien, Conn.: 15 November 1978), p. 28.

> blacks and incidence

P. F. Venter, "Endometriosis," *South African Medical Journal,* 57(1980), pp. 894–99.

> blacks in South Africa

JAY GOLD and JOHN B. JOSIMOVICH, "Endometriosis," in *Gynecolgic Endocrinology*, third ed. (Hagerstown, Md.: Harper & Row, 1980), p. 431.

> more prevalent in blacks than thought

DONALD CHATMAN and ANNE WARD, "Endometriosis in Adolescents," *The Journal of Reproductive Medicine*, 27 #3(1982), p. 156.

> black teenagers

Lippincott Manual of Nursing, third ed. (Philadelphia: J. B. Lippincott Co., 1982), p. 549.

> rare in blacks

A. BRZEZINSKI et al., "Contribution to the Problem of the Etiology of Endometriosis," *Israel Medical Journal* 21(1962), pp. 5–6.

> in Israeli women

JUDY LEVER, *Pre-menstrual Tension* (New York: Bantam, 1982), p. 52.

> Orthodox Jewish taboos;
> menstruation and intercourse

KUNIO MIYAZAWA, "Incidence of Endometriosis," *Obstetrics and Gynecology*, 48 (October 1976), pp. 407–8.

> in Oriental women

15 *Prevention*

BARRY S. SCHIFRIN et al., "Teen-age Endometriosis," *American Journal of Obstetrics and Gynecology*, 116, #7, (1973), pp. 973–80.

genital abnormalities and predisposition

"Endometriosis: New Views, New Therapies," (round-table discussion in *Patient Care*, 12, no. 19 (Darien, Conn.: 15 November 1978), p. 27.

tampon acts as wick

V. E. DAVIS, "Menstrual Coitus and Endometriosis," letter, *Medical Journal of Australia*, 1, #12 (13 June 1981), pp. 648–49.

intercourse during menstruation

LUCIENNE LANSON, *From Woman to Woman* (New York: Knopf, 1981), pp. 109, 293–94.

intercourse to relieve menstrual cramping; menstrual extraction

"Endometriosis: New Views, New Therapies," p. 27.

intercourse and endometriosis

KATHRYN SCHROTENBOER and GENELL J. SUBAK-SHARPE, *Freedom from Menstrual Cramps* (New York: Pocket Books, 1981), p. 117.

⅔ to ¾ of women will have intercourse by 20 years of age

BARBARA SEAMAN and GIDEON SEAMAN, *Women and the Crisis in Sex Hormones* (New York: Bantam, 1979), p. 198.

endometriosis and IUD

LYNDA MADARAS and JANE PATTERSON, *Womancare* (New York: Avon, 1981), pp. 95, 205–6.

cervical cap developed for wear during menstruation; menstrual extraction

ROBERT W. KISTNER, "Endometriosis," in *Gynecology and Obstetrics*, ed. John Sciarra (Hagerstown, Md.: Harper & Row, 1980), p. 24, reprint.

therapeutic pregnancy

P. F. VENTER, "Endometriosis," *South African Medical Journal,* 57, 1980, p. 897.

pregnancy and prevention

ELTON KESSEL, "Menstrual Regulation," in *Birth Control,* ed. Malcolm Potts and Pouru Bhiwandiwala (Baltimore: University Park Press, 1979), pp. 187–89.

menstrual extraction

MALCOLM POTTS, "Bi-cycle and Tri-cycle Pills," *IPPF Medical Bulletin.*

long-term Pill packets

DIANE KARNES, "How Nutrition Helped My Gynecological Problems," *Prevention,* August 1975, pp. 114–18.

nutrition and

16 Leeches and Laudanum: Grandmother and You

MME. VEUVE BOIVIN and A. DUGES, *A Practical Treatise on the Diseases of the Uterus* (London, 1834), pp. 94–97, 190–91, 496–97.

feminine health in nineteenth century

FREDERICK HOLLICK, *The Diseases of Woman, Their Causes and Cure Familiarly Explained; With Practical Hints for Their Prevention and for the Preservation of Female Health,* 49th ed. (New York: T. W. Strong, 1849), pp. 144–45, 176–77.

feminine health in nineteenth century

WALTER C. TAYLOR, *A Physician's Counsels to Woman in Health and Disease* (W. J. Holland & Co., 1871), pp. 296–97, 320–23.

feminine health in nineteenth century

JOHN MAUBRAY, *The Female Physician Containing All the Diseases Incident to That Sex, in Virgins, Wives, and Widows* (Bible & Ball in St. Paul's Church Yard, 1724), p. 387.

feminine health in eighteenth century

BARBARA EHRENREICH and DEIRDRE ENGLISH, *Complaints and Disorders: The Sexual Politics of Sickness.* Glass Mountain Pamphlet #2. (Old Westbury, N.Y.: The Feminist Press, 1973), p. 19.

childbirth mortality rates, 1915

Index

Abortion, 168
Adenomyosis, 15–17, 23, 42,
  130–32
Adolescents, xv–xvi, 25, 31, 63,
  119–25, 156–57
  black, 149
  pregnant, 162
  tampons, 160
Adrenal glands
  estrogen, 127, 129
American Fertility Society, 49, 56
Amniocentesis
  spread of endometriosis, 14
Appendix, 101
Arquembourg, Pierre, 20

Backache, 29
Ballweg, Mary Lou, 120, 142
Behrman, Dr. S. J., 96–98
Biopsy, 72, 153
  adolescents, 124
Birth control, 7, 180
  diaphragm, 162. *See also*
    Contraception
Black women, 39, 147–50, 154
Blood
  system, 23, 115, 120

Bowel
  endometriosis, 113–14
Breast cancer, 8
  estrogen, 24
  the Pill, 165
Brzezinski, Dr. A., 150

Caesarian section, 164
  spread of endometriosis, 14
Cancer, 41
  benign, 22–24, 156
  breast, 140, 165
  cells, 19, 20
  DES, 79
  differs from endometriosis,
    23–24
  estrogen replacement therapy
    (ERT), 128
  ovarian, 112–13, 154, 165
  rate, 84
  X-ray, 108
Career Woman's Disease, 133–45
Castration
  ovaries, 95, 96, 104
  X-rays, 109
Cervical cap, 162–63
Cervix, 97, 162

Cervix (continued)
  cauterizing, 98
  endometriosis of, 67
  laser surgery, 103-4
  surgical procedures, 164
Chalmers, J. A., M.D., 11, 67, 109
Chatman, Dr. Donald L., xv, xvi,
    121, 149
Childbearing
  and endometriosis, 154
  late, 138
"Chocolate" cysts, 72-73
Classification, 49-51
  body types, 133-34
Cleary, Edward, 87
Complications
  rare, 112-16
Contraception, 180
  adolescent, 25
  Jewish women, 151
  natural, 7
  oral, 165
Cost
  Danocrine, 87, 89
  insurance companies, 94, 101
  office procedures, 67
Cul-de-sac, 29, 42, 67, 99, 113
Cysts, 5, 8, 23, 27
  "chocolate," 72-73
  ovarian, 39, 41, 42-43

D&C (dilation and curettage), 32,
    68, 72, 163, 164
Danazol, 56, 85-86, 90-91, 97, 142,
    169, 170
  dosage, 89
  side effects (chart), 88
Danocrine, 86, 87
  cost, 89
Depo-Provera, 83-84, 108
DES (Diethyl-Stilbestrol), 79, 83
Diagnostic procedures, 64-65
Diet, 128, 129
Dilation and curettage, See D&C
Diverticulitis, 40-41
Dmowski, Dr. W. P., 84, 129

Drake, Dr. Terrance S., 55-56
Dysmenorrhea, 12, 27-29, 55, 63,
    122, 176-77
  PSN surgery, 100
Dyspareunia, 29

Ectopic pregnancy, 40
Ekwempu, Dr. C. C., 148
Endometrial implants
  chart, 49
  endoscopy, 48
  hormones, 82
  spread, 37
Endometrial tissue, 18, 39
  in Fallopian tubes, 40
  removal, 168
  spread of, 163
  surgical scars and, 14, 164
Endometriomas (large cysts), 42,
    73, 74, 105
  hormones, 82
  of ovary, 97
Endometriosis
  adenomyosis, 15-17
  adolescents, xv-xvi, 9, 12,
    119-25
  bowel, 113-14
  childbearing, 154
  defined, 5, 19
  differs from cancer, 23-24
  diagnostic procedures, 64-65
  genetic predisposition theory,
    24-25
  hormonal imbalance theory,
    21-22
  history, 173-81
  immunologic theory, 19-20
  infertility, 7, 20
    leading cause, 9, 46
  lung, 114
  menstruation and, 5-6
    retrograde theory, 10-12
  navel, 114
  nosocomial infection, 13-15
  ovarian, 112-13
  percent of women affected, 19,
    152, 154

race, xv, 109, 146–54
radiation, 108–11
retroverted uterus, 12
scar, 15
sites (chart), 115–16
symptoms, 22, 26–43
transformation theory, 22–24
transplantation theory, 12–13
Endometriosis Association
    (Milwaukee), 119, 120, 124,
    142
address, 125
Endometriosis externa, 30–31, 42,
    130, 131
Jewish women, 150–51
study of Hausa/Fulani women,
    148
Endometriosis interna
    (adenomyosis), 16, 30, 42,
    130
study of Hausa/Fulani women,
    148
symptoms, 130–31
treatment, 131
Endometrium, 3, 5
Enovid, 82, 83
Episiotomy, 164
spread of endometriosis, 14–15
ERT. *See* Estrogen replacement
    therapy
Estrogen, 3, 21, 57, 77, 83, 105, 129
after hysterectomy, 106, 107
and cancers, 24
in DES, 79
in the Pill, 7
menopause, 127
side effects, 81
Estrogen replacement therapy
    (ERT), 128–29, 130

Fallopian tubes, 10, 40, 42, 54, 97,
    157, 161, 163, 168
appear open, 18, 30
dysmenorrhea, 12
hysterogram, 48
laparoscopy, 68–69
PID, 149

retrograde menstruation, 11,
    120
Rubin test, 39, 48
USN, 100
FDA. *See* Food and Drug
    Administration, U.S.
Feminine Forever, 144
Fertility, 7, 105, 179
adolescents, 162
Fertility and Sterility, 134
Fibroid tumors, 7, 8, 131
estrogen, 83
Follicle, 54
cyst, 42
menopause, 127
Follicle-stimulating hormones.
    See FSH
Food and Drug Administration,
    U.S. (FDA), 56, 81
Depo-Provera, 84
Fourestier, Gladu, 66
Fox, C. A., 160, 162
Frank, Drs. Arthur and Stuart, 63
Freedom from Menstrual Cramps,
    27, 63
From Woman to Woman, 161,
    168
FSH (follicle-stimulating
    hormone), 21, 85, 127

Genetic predisposition, 24–25
adolescents, 121
Genital abnormalities, 157–59
Gifford-Jones ,W., 94
Glands
adrenal, 127
hypothalamus, 21
lymph, 12, 23
pituitary, 21
Gold, Jay, M.D., 99, 134
Goldman, Emma, 180
Goldstein, Dr. Donald, 121
adolescent study, 123
Gonorrhea, 43
*Good Housekeeping Family
    Health and Medical Guide,*
    126

Greenblatt, Dr. Robert, 28
Gynecological Endocrinology,
    99, 134, 150

Harrison, K. A., 148
Harrison, Michelle, M.D., 15, 147
Harvard Medical School, 8, 10
    Countway Medical Library,
        xviii
Hausa/Fulani (Nigeria)
    study of, 148
Hernia, 41
Hiroshima, 109, 110
Historical highlights, 171–72
Hollick, Dr. Frederick, 175–77,
    181
"Hormonal Aspects of
    Endometriosis, The," 79
Hormones, 8, 165, 169
    follicale-stimulating (FSH), 21
    imbalance theory, 21–22
    lutinizing (LH), 21
    menopause, 127–29
    treatment, 77–91
Huhner test (postcoital), 47
Human Pathology, 14, 112
Hysterectomy, 31–32, 78, 93–95,
    106–7, 131
    radical, 105–6, 129
Hysterogram (X-ray test), 48
Hysteroscopy, 67

Iffy, Dr. L., 40
Immunity, 19
    immunologic theory, 19–20, 23
Index Medicus, xviii, 146
Infertility, 7, 9, 44–58, 154
    immune studies, 20
    percent, 30, 44
    prostaglandins, 55
    radiation, 110
    symptom, 29, 30
Intercourse. *See* Sexual
    intercourse
International Fertility Research
    Program, 6

International Health Foundation
    (Geneva), 166
International Journal of Fertility,
    40
International Planned Parenthood,
    110
Intrauterine device. *See* IUD
Israel, 150, 151
IUD, 7–8, 25, 74, 162–63

Janovski, Dr. Nikolas, 162
Japan
    hospital study, 109–10
Japanese women, 153
Jewish women, 150–52
    contraceptives, 151
Johns Hopkins Medical Center,
    138, 152
Johns Hopkins University, 164
Josimovich, John, M.D., 99, 134

Kalk, Dr. H., 66
Karman, Harvey, 167
Karnes, Diane, 57, 91, 114–15,
    169, 170
Keith, Carolyn, 120
Kessel, Elton, 168
Kistner, Dr. Robert W., 8, 27, 29,
    40, 62, 73, 97, 104, 108,
    112–13, 135
    adolescents, 121
    danazol, 89
    estrogen, 106
    hormonal treatment, 84
    immunity, 19
    infertility, 8, 54
    retrograde menstruation, 10
Kobe Hospital (Japan), 153
Kung bush women, 6

Lamb, Dr. Karen, 142
Lanson, Dr. Lucienne, 161, 162
Laparoscope, 8
    origin, 66
Laparoscopy, 10, 25, 35, 63, 66–72,
    122, 141, 146

adolescents, 124, 157
black women, 147, 149
diagnostic, 95
Laparotomy, 99, 150, 152
spread of endometriosis, 14
Laser, 103–4
LH (lutinizing hormone), 21, 85, 127
Lippincott Manual of Nursing, 149
Lloyd, Frank P., 149
Lungs, 13, 114
Lutinizing hormones. *See* LH
Lydia Pinkham (tonic), 173, 180
Lymph
    system, 23, 115, 120

Mademoiselle, 27, 63
Mal(e)practice: How Doctors Manipulate Women, 15, 75, 94, 107
Malinak, Dr. Russell, 82, 105, 129, 141, 160, 161
Manganiello, Dr. Paul, 16, 63, 87, 107, 130, 140, 163
Marik, Dr. Jaroslav, 16, 45, 67
Masturbation, 161
Mayo Clinic, 173
Medicaid, 89
Medical Journal of Australia, 160
Medical Letter, 86
Medical World News, 55
Memoria Casus Rari, 175
Menarche (first menstrual period), 6, 157
Mendelsohn, Robert, M.D., 15, 75, 94, 107, 144
Menopause, 6, 64, 77, 92–93, 108, 126–32
    early, 106–7, 129–30
    hormones, 127–29
    osteoporosis, 129
Menorrhagia (excessive flow), 30
Menstrual extraction, 167–68
Menstruation
    excessive, 30
    process of, 3

retrograde, 10, 12, 120, 122
spot bleeding, 30
Metastasis, 12, 23
Michael Reese Hospital (Chicago), 70
Microsurgery, 102–4
Mikvah (ritual bath)
    Jewish women, 151
Motrin, 22, 55, 56, 63
Ms., 127

Navel
    endometriosis, 114
Nevada
    atomic test sites, 110
New England Journal of Medicine, 61
Nigeria, 17
    study, 167
Niles, Dr. Herbert, 79, 147, 149, 150
Nodules, 42, 98
Nora, Dr. Ernest, 57
Nosocomial infection (accidental implantation), 13–15
Nutrition, 155, 168–70

Obstetrics and Gynecology, 109
Obstetrics & Gynecology Annual 1981, 84
Oophorectomy
    bilateral, 129
Orgasm, 161
Oriental women, 109, 152–54
Osteoporosis, 129
Osterholm, Dr. Michael, 159
Our Bodies, Ourselves, 120'
Ovary
    cancer, 165
    castration, 95, 96, 104
    cysts, 73
    egg release, 21
    endometrioma, 97
    endometriosis, 112–13, 154
    estrogen, 24
    removal, 129

Pain
  menstrual, 27–28
Patient Care, 16, 28, 82, 104, 141
Pelvic inflammatory disease. *See*
  PID
Penis, 161
Periods
  number of, 6
Personality, 136–38
Physician's Counsels to a Woman,
  in Health and Disease, A,
  178
PID (pelvic inflammatory
  disease), 38–39, 141, 165
  black women, 147, 148
Pill, the, 7, 25, 58, 63, 78–79,
  81–82, 122, 157
  beneficial aspects, 164–66
  death rate, 83
Planned Parenthood. *See*
  International Planned
  Parenthood
Pogash, Carol, 45, 46, 47–48
Potts, Dr. Malcolm, 6, 8, 139, 165,
  166
Pregnancy, 167
  in developed countries, 6
  in primitive tribes, 6
  menstruation and, 6, 7
  rates, hormonal, 85
  resembling, 8
Premarin, 106
Presacral Neurectomy. *See* PSN
Prevention, 155–70
Prevention, 57, 91, 114, 169
Primitive tribes, 6
Progesterone, 3, 21, 54, 57, 83
Prostaglandins, 21, 55–56
  inhibitor, 63, 122, 124
    adolescents, 157
    severe cramps, 22
Pseudomenopause, 77, 97
Pseudopregnancy, 77, 78–85, 86,
  97
PSN (Presacral Neurectomy),
  99–100, 101
Puberty, 9

Race, xv, 146–54
  Orientals, 153
  study, 109
Radiation
  atomic bomb
    Hiroshima, 110
  castration, 110
  therapy, 108–11
Rakoff, Dr. Abraham, 16, 42
Rectum
  bleeding, 30
Recurrence, 107
Redbook, 45
Relman, Dr. Arnold, 61
Retrograde menstruation, 10, 12,
  120, 122
  suction, 161
Rock, Dr. John, 138, 152, 160
Rodale, 169
  Woman's Encyclopedia of
    Health and Natural
    Healing, 126
Rothschild-Hadassah University
  Hospital (Jerusalem), 150
Rubin test, 39, 48, 164

Sampson, John, 10, 12, 22
  retrograde menstruation, 11
Sanger, Margaret, 180
Schneider, Dr. George T., 19, 20,
  108, 147
Schrotenboer, Dr. Kathryn, 27
Sciarra, John, 56
Seaman, Barbara and Gideon, 81,
  82, 128, 170
Sexual intercourse
  during menstruation, 151,
    160–62
  survey, 160
Sheldon, William, 133
Short, Dr. Roger, 7
Second opinion, 94–95
Socioeconomic status, 138–40,
  141, 148
Somatotypes, 133, 134–35
South African Medical Journal,
  148, 166

Sperm count, 46–47
State University of New York
    Downstate Medical Center,
    76
Sturgis, Somers, 128
Surgery, 78, 92–107, 169–70
    laser, 103–4
    radical, 104–7
Symptoms, 26–43
    adolescents, 156–57
    similar, 38–43
    sites, 35

Taboo
    menstrual, 160
Tampons, 151
    versus sanitary pads, 159–60
Taylor, W. J., 178–80
Teenagers. *See* Adolescents
Time-Line, 142–43
Toxic shock syndrome, 159

Ultrasound, 74–76
    pregnant women, 75
Umbilicus (navel), 41
Upjohn Laboratories, 84
Urinalysis, 37
USN (Uterosacral Neurectomy),
    100–101
Uterosacral Neurectomy. *See*
    USN
Uterus
    accidental implantation, 14–15
    adenomyosis, 15–17, 130
    "boggy," 130
    cancer, 165
    endometrial fragments outside,
        11
    estrogen, 24
    hysterogram, 48

monkey experiments, 11
prostaglandins in, 21
pseudopregnancy, 97
retroverted, 12, 54, 122, 161, 180
suspending, 98
tipped, 12
USN surgery, 100–101

Vaccines, 155
Vagina
    surgical procedures, 164
van Keep, Dr., 166
Venter, Dr. P. F., 148, 149, 161,
    166
Visualization, 153
Vitamins, 169

Ward, Anne B., M.D., xv–xvi, 70,
    121, 149
Weed, John, 20
Wiedmann, Dr., 175
*What Every Woman Should
    Know About
    Hysterectomy*, 94
Wilson, Dr. Robert, 144
Winthrop Laboratories, 86, 87,
    142, 154
Woman in Residence, A, 15, 147
Womancare, 16, 23, 47, 66, 107,
    168
*Woman's Encyclopedia of Health
    and Natural Healing*
    (Rodale), 126
*Women and the Crisis in Sex
    Hormones*, 81–82, 128, 170
World Health Organization, 165

X-rays, 76
    castration, 109, 110, 111
    See also Radiation